BIG ARMS

AND

HOW TO DEVELOP THEM

(Original Version, Restored)

by

BOB HOFFMAN

"The world's leading physical director" - Editor in Chief of Strength and Health Magazine

Originally published by Strength & Health Publishing Company, 1939

PUBLISHED BY O'Faolain Patriot L L C, Copyright 2012

info@physicalculturebooks.com

ISBN-13: 978-1469930930

ISBN-10: 1469930935

Published in the United States of America

To Order More Copies Visit: PhysicalCultureBooks.com

FOREWORD

There is more interest in arm development than in any other part of the body. A large part of our correspondence is from those ambitious body builders who wish to develop larger arms. In spite of the great number of articles Strength and Health Magazine has contained in the past concerning advice to develop the arms, readers never seem to obtain enough.

At the senior national A. A. U. championships July 4th this year in Chicago, a number of men had scarcely been introduced, or introduced themselves, until they said, " Say, Bob, when are you going to have another article on arm development? It's been six months since the last one appeared. All the members of our club are interested in increasing their arm size and would like to receive more instruction and training hints upon building the arms."

I mentioned the fact that there have been an average of two articles yearly in Strength and Health Magazine covering all phases of arm development—with dumbells, cables, bar bells, lifting, balancing and tumbling. Isn't that enough?

" We never get enough," was the reply. " We'd rather have bigger arms that anything we know of."

From what I have heard and seen I believe that the opinion of the young man in Chicago is not the exception but the rule. I've been present at hundreds of weight lifting and strength shows, and the crowd is always eager to have the leading strength athletes show their arms. At Cuba this last winter, scores of requests were made for Tony Terlazzo, Gord Venables, John Grimek or myself to display our arms.

I remember one day on the beach at Miami (don't think I spend my time down there under a palm tree—it was my first visit to the southern tropical city, and I worked nearly every minute I was there) overhearing a conversation. John

Grimek was with us and the conversation from a nearby group ran like this: " Look at the arms that guy has. Wonder what he does to get them! Must be a wrestler."

When I look at John Grimek I see his arms—they're wonderful enough—but I see much more than that: A powerful, symmetrical physique, with column-like neck, broad shoulders, huge rounded chest, exceptionally narrow waist, powerful thighs and extraordinary calves. He's physical perfection in itself. But the men and women on the sands of Miami saw only the arms.

I remember another day I was standing among a crowd of people on the streets of York as a circus parade was passing. Several men called out from the circus wagons, " Hey, guy, you with the muscles, or you with the big arms! What are you, a wrestler? Come out to the circus and see us. We want to talk to you." Out of a crowd of some thousands of people they saw the Grimek arms, and it didn't take such sharp eyes to see them either, for they are most conspicuous.

Hundreds of similar experiences have proven that people —the body builders and the uninitiated alike—like, crave for and admire big arms. In my opinion the arms are not nearly as important as other muscle groups of the body— not more than one-tenth as strong as the legs or the back; but people always have and always will prefer big arms. Might as well try to transform night into day as change the opinion that the strength of a man is denoted by the size and development of the arms.

Everyone wants big arms. And this book is my Answer to that desire. It is the most complete arm development book ever ollered to the strength and development-seeking public. It contains more good, tried and proven, result- producing exercises, and a great many others which are completely new or little known, than have ever been included in a single volume. I have urged those who receive this book to practice an all-round training or body-building program for strength inside and out. Better operating organs and better internal processes are the result of all- around training. Bigger, stronger arms are developed when all the muscles are strengthened.

This general body-building program, with a certain amount of specialization upon arm development, should produce for the conscientious follower of the exercising system this book includes striking-appearing, admiration- creating, really powerful and large-sized arms.

Follow the advice and the exercises this book contains and you'll be proud of the results obtained and can take your place among that small group of powerful-armed men who are noted for their strength and development. I wish all who read this book, and follow the advice and instruction it contains, the best of success in realizing their desires for BIG ARMS.

The Author.

CONTENTS

"Let Me Feel Your Muscle"

"LET me feel your muscle." If you have advanced reasonably far in the acquisition of strength and development, and that request or demand were made of you, what muscle would you permit the curious person to feel? In perhaps 999 cases out of a thousand the Biceps would be the muscle group displayed. In the minds of most men and boys, the arm is always thought of as the muscle. And the front of the arm, the Biceps, is the part of the arm that is usually revealed or felt.

There is something fascinating about the development of the upper arms. Although there is no advanced weight man who does not realize that the upper arms play the least important part in elevating a great poundage overhead, there is probably not one of them who does not show more interest in the development of the muscles of the arm than those of any other part of the body. I don't believe there is a man anywhere who would not accept the gift of a larger pair of arms if he could get them. But they can not be had as a gift. Hard work, as we will relate in subsequent chapters, is required to produce the best arms. The more work, the greater variety of proper exercises, intelligently practiced, the finer will be the resulting development of the arm.

It's the aim of the majority of physical culturists to obtain big arms. The bigger the better, they believe. The young enthusiast who desires the maximum in strength and development finds it much more convenient to display the new muscles of the upper arm to his friends than the muscles of any other group.

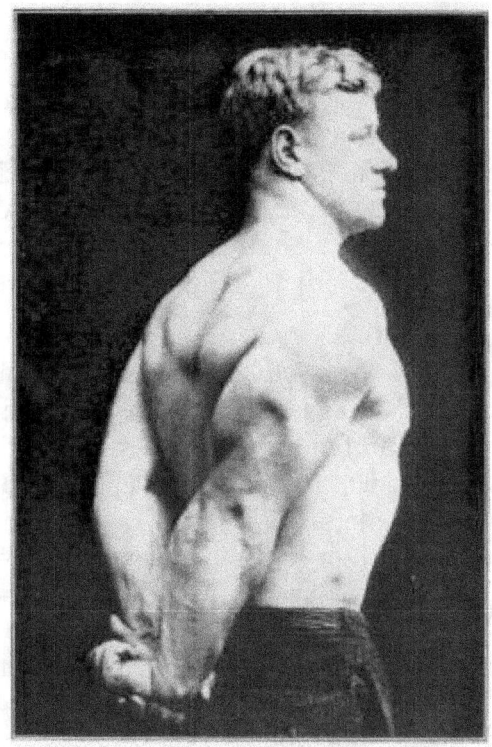

Joe Nordquest, one of the most powerful men ever developed in America. His arms were 19 inches.

There are more than 4,000,000,000 muscular fibres in the body. Old and young, frail and strong, all have the same number of muscular fibres. The only difference between the thin, eleven-inch arm of the undeveloped young man and the powerful, swelling, beautifully-moulded arm of the strength champions—the men who possess the greatest strength and development; men like John Grimek, Steve Stanko or Dave Mayor—is the size and development of the arms. The fibres through constant use have grown in bulk, power and shapeliness and a really big arm results.

More than half of these 4,000,000,000 muscular fibres are located in the lower limbs. Of the remaining half, less than one-eighth would be in the arms, and of these approximately one-sixth are located in the Biceps group. According to this line of reasoning the Biceps would be about one one-hundredth of the muscular bulk of the body. The powerful lower limbs are usually ten times as strong as the arms. The world's record in the back lift is 4,300 pounds, the world's record in the harness lift, in which the legs supply most of the power, is 3,600 pounds. While men have supported over 5,000 pounds on their extended lower limbs, the world's record in the two hands press is 317 pounds.

In spite of these facts, well known to all advanced body builders, far more effort is placed back of building mighty arms than is spent in the development of any other part of the body. You can test the truth of what I have written if you wish. Just ask the average man or boy who believes that he is strong to show you his muscle and invariably he will roll up his sleeve and show you the muscle of the upper arm. Not once in a thousand times would a man ask you to feel his back or legs, when you are interested in measuring his strength. The desire to obtain bigger upper arms is paramount in the minds of most body culturists.

Although all men of might and muscle, all the leading lifters do not have big arms, everyone will want them Human nature is the result of untold thousands of generations of humanity who have lived upon this earth throughout the ages. Might as well try to change a leopard's spots as to try to alter human nature. Since the majority of people will always believe that the size, appearance and hardness of the upper arm, its development, is the best way to estimate the power of the body, most physical culturists or body builders will be more interested in developing the arms than any other part of the anatomy.

Therefore, I am writing this book for the legion of men who want big arms. It will contain the best tried and proven information about building the arms. I hope it will serve as a complete text book on the development of the arms from the point where the upper end of the Biceps and Triceps is fastened to the Humerus, to the other extremity in the complex assembly of the hands.

Although it is my intention to endeavor to compile by far the most complete book on developing the arms ever published, I do wish to warn all who read this book and put into practice the training information it contains not to permit the great desire to obtain a big upper arm to cause you to neglect the development of the remainder of the body. You should strive for all around physical excellence. Big arms are generally the result of all around training. A moderate amount of specializing; in arm development should be sufficient to bring them to outstanding size, strength and proportions. You could not expect to use a Mack truck tire on a Ford or other light car. Neither could you expect to build a seventeen inch arm upon a 120 pound body. It's essential that a bigger body be built, so that bigger arms may be obtained.

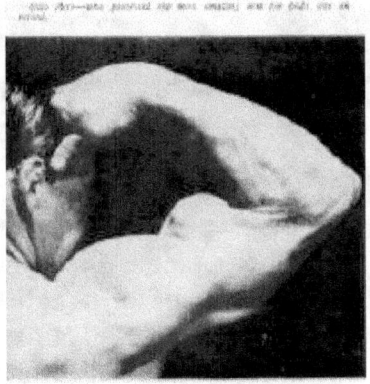

History has proven that the men who have owned and now are famed for their magnificent arms are men who possessed the best all around developments. A powerful body which is the result of all around physical training has helped them build their big upper arms. For to build the arms to their limit it is necessary to handle heavy weights.

The handling of heavy weights brings into play other muscles of the body, builds the power of the internal organs, improves the function of the glands, benefits digestion, assimilation, elimination, creates appetite, favors the little known process of metabolism which prepares the food taken into the body for later assimilation. Heavy exercise improves circulation, speeds up respiration, breaks down tissue which is replaced by the healthy blood stream. Big arms are better obtained as one of the products of all around training.

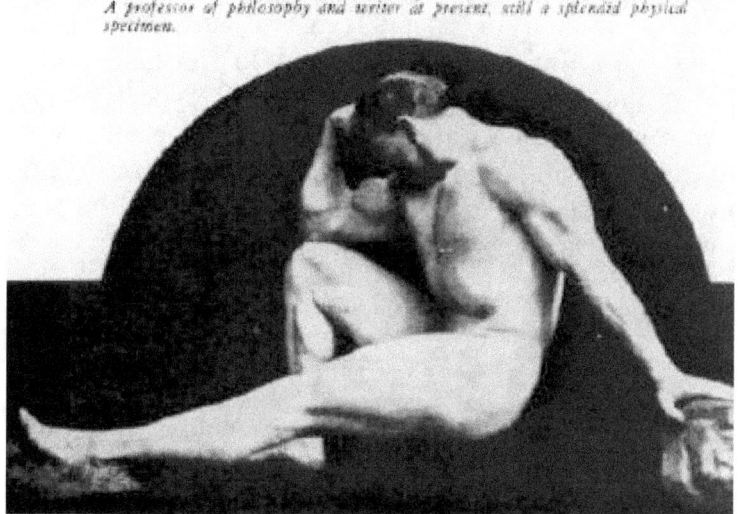

George Hackenschmidt, world's lifting and wrestling champion of 1908. A professor of philosophy and writer at present, still a splendid physical specimen.

The men today who possess the finest developed arms, those which stretch the tape to its greatest girth, are America's strongest men. Of the strength athletes of today, Dave Mayor, heavyweight national lifting champion of 1937, has the biggest muscular arms in the world, i9^1/-> inches. Dave weighs 265 pounds, and it's natural that he should have a bigger arm than a man who weighs less, but Steve Stanko, America's strongest weight lifter at present, has an arm rapidly approaching 19 inches in girth. At a height of approximately six feet, Steve is a real powerhouse.

He has a great development in every part of his body and his huge, well-developed arms are not the result of specialization in Biceps development but of all around training. A moderate amount of special training would increase the size of his arms by at least a full inch and bring them up to the small group of nineteen inch armed men, I believe.

Although John Grimek, world famous for his marvellously developed physique, is not a huge man as big men go—he was Heavyweight National Champion in 1936, a member of the Olympic team, hoisting the highest American lifting total at the Berlin Olympics—he has an eighteen inch arm at any time. His arms have measured 18V2 inches, when his bodyweight was a bit higher than the 190 pounds where he normally keeps it. When he weighs over two hundred, as he has at times, his arm is naturally bigger than when he contends in the 181 pound class as he did to become a member of the world's championship team of 1938 which competed in Vienna, and to win the championship of North America that year.

The bigger men usually have the biggest arms. So if you wish an arm which is really outstanding you must increase the weight and development of your entire body. Don't fail to strive for all around development. Then a moderate amount of arm specialization methods such as I will offer in this book will bring your arms to the point where they will be outstanding for your height and weight. If you arc well developed at no, 120 or 150 pounds or less, you can obtain a development, an impressive appearing arm, which will be as large in proportion as the eighteen inch arms of the larger fellows. Little Firpo Lemma, the 112 pound U. S. champion and world's record holder, has a small arm, but one which is marvelously developed. It is not expected that a larger arm could be placed upon his small body.

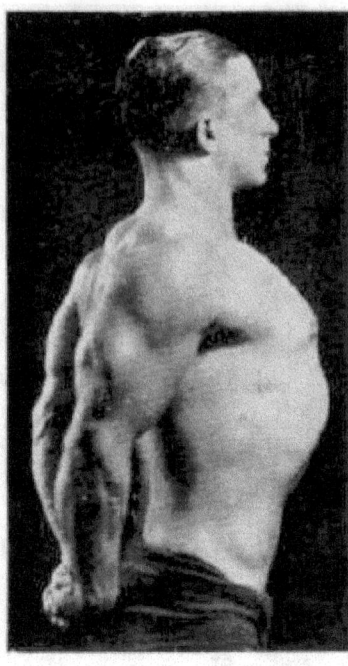

Muscular bulk is desirable, but as a general thing it includes considerable of adipose tissue which greatly adds to its bulk. One of the greatest strength athletes who ever lived—George Lurich, the Russian—had arms of only 15V2 inches, according to the best authorities. Yet he two arm jerked to arm's length overhead the great weight of 350 pounds. He has held the one arm jerk record for many years,—266 pounds. Lurich weighed 190 pounds, yet his record exceeds by many pounds the best attempts of men who outweighed him by as much as a hundred pounds.

A man must have bodyweight and great bulk over all his body if he desires to acquire an arm comparing favorably with the largest of the great old timers' arms. Louis Gyr, considered by many to be the strongest man who ever lived, is credited with a pair of arms which measured 22 inches when flexed. It is natural that his arms should be large for he possessed great strength in all parts of his body and always weighed over 300 pounds. His training mate, Horace Barre, while not as famous for his strength, principally owing to his lethargic disposition, retiring nature and dislike to extend himself or show himself before a crowd, is not so well known, but those who knew him well attest to the fact that he had arms as large as Cyr and many believe as great all around strength.

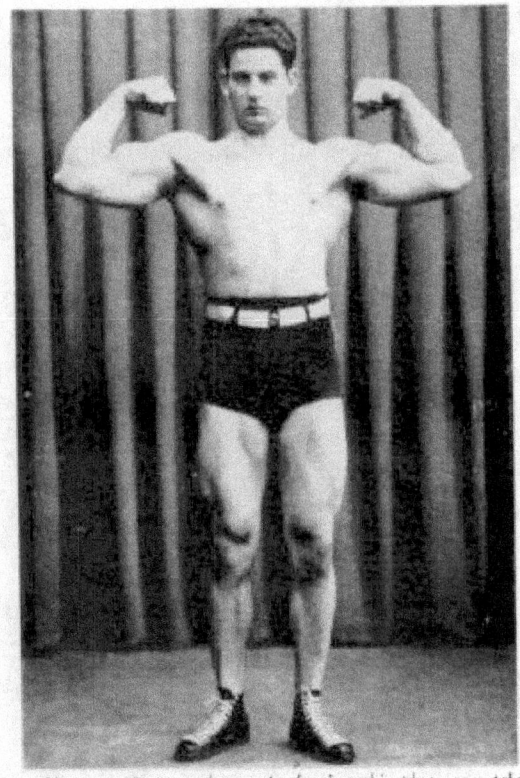

Dave Mayor at 19 years of age. At the time this photo was taken he weighed 220 pounds and his arm was 18 inches. Later it stretched the tape to a full 19½ inches as he gained in weight

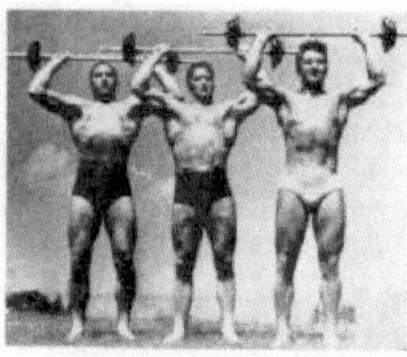

The two hands
military press.

Stanley Zbyszko, well known as the man who won the world's professional wrestling championship at the age of 57, always had phenomenal arms. As a young man he had an arm girth of nearly 21 inches. A bit later in life his arm measured 22 inches. These are the two largest arms of which we have an authentic record, although Ivan Sanakov, a Russian strength athlete, had an arm which measured 21V2 inches. Louis Uni, better known as Appollon, the French strong man and giant of the past, had enormous forearms and a Biceps which stretched the tape to 21 inches. At the age of 52, an age at which most men are thicker skinned and have some surplus tissue, he had an arm measurement of 22 inches.

Herman Corner, the South African German, and Charles Rigoulot, the great French professional champion and world's record holder, have the largest arms of the more recent professionals. Gorner is credited with a really muscular arm of 19 inches, which would compare favorably with the biggest of all time if it included the adipose tissue most of the bulky strong men possessed. Rigoulot's arm measurement exceeds 18 inches. The old time strong men were especially proud of their upper arm development as shown in the pictures for which they posed. The arms were nearly as conspicuous as the more than generous waist measurements of these old timers. A big man who has exercised and also possesses some adiposity will possess large arm measurements. The young man who has a moderate body weight and trains in such a manner that he avoids the oversize waistline, can not hope to equal the measurements of the men who are overweight. But he will have a much more attractive development.

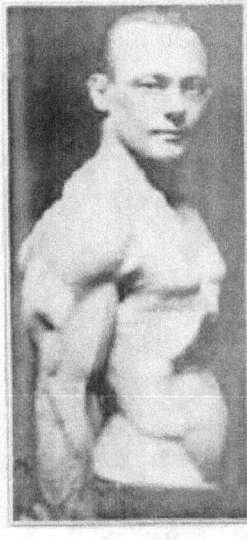

There are some men who desire only bulk, yet I would list shapeliness and strength well ahead of bulk. Quality of muscle coupled with outstanding proportions and fair size is much more to be desired than just a huge arm.

The largest arm in proportion to bodily weight of which I have ever heard was that of Joe Prada, who was an expert ring performer. He had a nearly 16 inch arm and weighed just 124 pounds. He carried upper arm development to the limit. He did all slow work on the rings and tied weights to his feet to provide progression. The same sort of resistance work could better be performed with the York Iron Boot. Prada also did considerable lifting but practiced only slow work with the weights, exercises which he could feel every inch of the way. His usual exercises were the bent press, side press—both performed with many repetitions—the one arm military press, two hands pressing both behind and in front of neck, the two hands curl, the rowing motion and holding weights out to the sides. He did a great deal of curling and pressing while seated upon a chair. He could curl more in proportion to weight than anyone on record. He made no attempt to develop his legs so was never able to obtain the limit in developing the power of his arms.

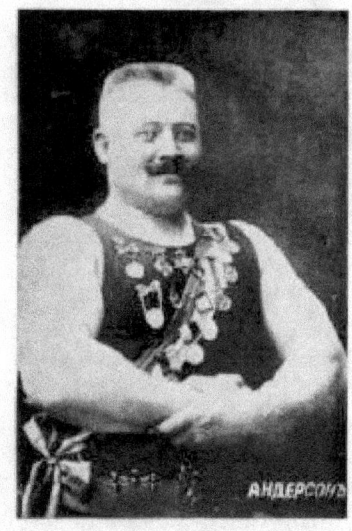

Ivan Sandou, Russian strength athlete who possessed an arm measuring 20½ inches.

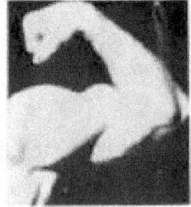

The powerful arm of Ronie Sandou, 1917 and 1920 United States champion (a measures 18½ inches.)

Another great ring performer was Victor Marcantoni, and although much larger and heavier than the average ring performer, there were feats he performed which few if any of his smaller and lighter rivals could achieve. He and his two partners also did hand to hand work and he was credited with a 220 pound press. He devoted considerable time to weight lifting and his arms were among the finest ever seen.

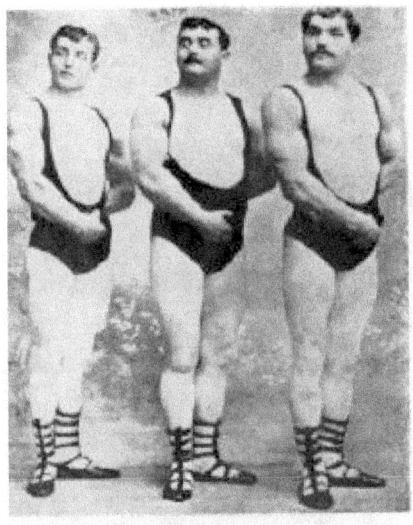

The would famous Saxon Trio, Arthur Saxon, the world's greatest one arm lifter, is shown at the right.

There was a British weight man who had a burning desire to obtain the greatest arm development on record for his bodyweight. He specialized in endless repetitions at one arm curling. He used very heavy poundages, permitting only a few repetitions with each exercise, but spent long hours each training day working his arms. And this man, T. W. Clarke, was rewarded by attaining a pair of 16% inch arms at his bodyweight of 154 pounds.

Arthur Saxon, the greatest one arm lifter who ever lived, had fine arms—although not large in proportion to his great strength. They seldom measured over 17 inches. Eugene Sandow laid claim to huge arms, at times publishing their girth as 19 inches. But in the same book he offered his measurements as taken by the late Dr. Sargent, and the average measurement was given as 16 1/2 inches (16.1 left;

16.9 right)—far less than 19, but huge, nevertheless, for Sandow weighed around 180 pounds.

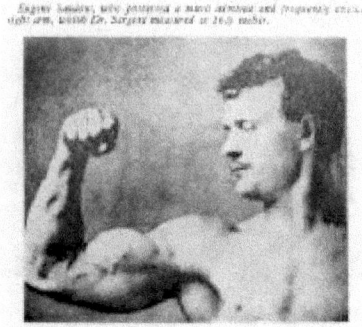

Eugene Sandow, who possessed a most sinuous and frequently curled right arm, which Dr. Sargent measured at 16.9 inches.

Hercules, Ajax, Mars, Achilles, Hector

This book would not be complete without some reference to the sculptural masterpieces of the past. These old artists have glorified .the strength and physiques of the athletes of their day. The ancient masters in many cases spent their entire lives reproducing in marble, bronze and on canvas the figures of the beautifully-formed women and the strong men of their day— immortalized them so that we who live thousands of years later can enjoy seeing the beauty and the strength of the physiques represented.

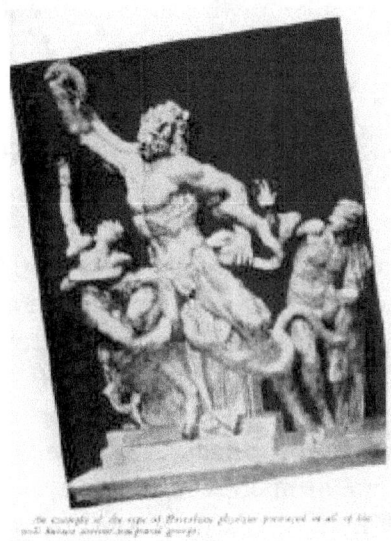

An example of the type of Grecian physique pictured in all of the well-known ancient sculptural groups.

Posterity has received the legacy left by these representatives of a great people of the past. The artists and sculptors of that distant day have proven their love of and belief in all that is beautiful, strong and healthy. Throughout the ages history has repeated itself. Macedonia, Sparta, Carthage, Greece and Rome each took their turn at ruling the world, until dissipation and a love of, and indulgence in, luxury took the place of physical exercise with its resulting strength creating and good health building. A nation remains strong and virile as long as its people strive to excel physically. When the time came that they were willing to rely upon the muscles of slaves as did the great nations which fell in the past, or are willing to be served entirely by modern conveniences as we have today, then that nation falls. In the past, the world leaders were overrun by savage nations—barbarians as far as the arts were concerned, but men who still believed in physical strength and physical ability.

That's one of the paramount reasons for dedicating my life to encouraging the men and women of our nation to continue to strive to better themselves physically. In many other countries of the world there is physical training, usually with government supervision—enforced physical training. This makes the dictator ruled nations strong. We may not subscribe to their theories of government, but we must admit that their rulers are building a strong, virile race of people—cannon fodder, if you prefer to phrase it in that manner, but men who will conquer the world unless we of this country and of other democratic nations continue to keep ourselves strong through physical training. Strength begets courage and confidence; strength is the best means to peace. And our nation will lead the world just as long as the younger generation and each succeeding generation continues to retain an interest in their physical selves, their appearance, strength, and are willing to work toward the end of excelling physically.

Just as long as a race of people or a nation excel physically, are really strong, healthy and beautiful, its men and women will be mentally and spiritually strong and beautiful. And just as sure as death and taxes, when a race of people or a nation succumb to a willingness to indulge their bodies in empty ease, idleness, dissipation or even vicious licentiousness, when they reach the point of believing or imagining that they can continue to retain or develop red-blooded, strong, virile bodies by substituting vitriolic dissipation for dynamic exercise, there is bound to be but one result—complete failure and collapse of their civilization; the conquering of their country by stronger, more ambitious, more courageous men, who so organize their lives that they strive industriously to be stronger and healthier, that they live simple, wholesome lives and keep themselves at the peak physically. A close study of modern and ancient history, the history of man as man and woman as woman, has many times proven this to be true.

America is strong because we are only a generation or two removed from hard-working, simple-living, courageous, ambitious pioneers. Now that our mode of living has changed with many modern conveniences, labor-saving devices, short hours of work, it is imperative to keep our nation at the head of the parade of nations; that we make up for the hard work and simple living of our strong ancestors by spending some time at physical training and the living of lives not too different from those which helped our ancestors make this nation great.

We can take an important lesson from the people of the past. More than ever in the world's history, except, perhaps, in the days of ancient Greece, when every man and woman strove to possess a sound, beautiful body and an active, intelligent mind, we have a race of people interested in their health and their strength. Everything runs in cycles, and now it is becoming decidedly unfashionable to be fat, skinny, round-shouldered, hump-backed, or to bear any other of the physical marks which are proof of ignorance, laziness, or both. We have a great many men today who compare more than favorably with the subjects who posed for the ancient masterpieces. It is natural that we should, for we have more people, more men who are interested in excelling physically; we have better training methods and better equipment.

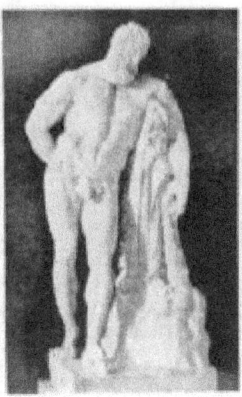

The Farnese Hercules. A early Herculean type. The marble piece was made more than two thousand years ago, and a doubt to be above any other statue of its kind, that it is doubtless it took a most rare head. It is believed that in certain unappraised the sculptures of our noblest portrayed to attributes his own ideal of what the most robust physique should be, when completely developed.

It has been my pleasure recently to serve as a judge or official in some capacity at a number of "Mr. America" contests, and I am more sure than ever that never before in the world's history were there so many outstanding, beautifully-developed, handsome examples of masculine perfection as we have at present. I have talked to artists, sculptors, men and women who have lived -to a great measure revelling in the masterpieces of the past. They see our men of the present and feel in the case of many of these models that no ancient master ever had a better model, a greater inspiration. It's more than doubtful if a man ever lived who possesses the all-around development and beauty of physique which has been developed by John Grimek. His physique, immortalized by the artists of the present, will prove to the men and women of the future generations that we of the 20th century rank more than favorably in physical excellence with the men of the past who flourished during the artistic periods of centuries ago.

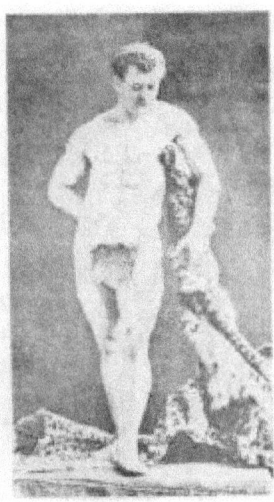

The sculptural masterpieces which have been bequeathed to us by these long dead artists personify superhuman strength, development and massive proportions. Of these the Farnese Hercules is one of the best known. The male figure depicted by the creator of the Farnese Hercules is shown with every muscle tensed—not a natural condition, 'tis true, but one which illustrates to the lover of the powerful masculine physique the tremendous development of which man is capable. John Grimek and Tony Massimo, I believe, are the two best modern representatives of this Herculean type. Sandow has been shown in the Farnese Hercules pose, but, weighing as he did just 181 pounds, he is not as huge and powerful as the truly Herculean Farnese Hercules.

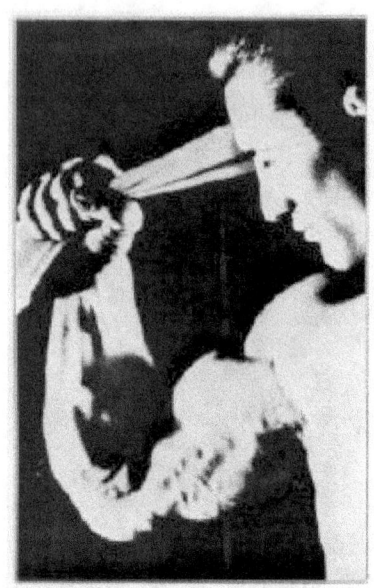

One of the most Herculean of modern men, Tony Massimo

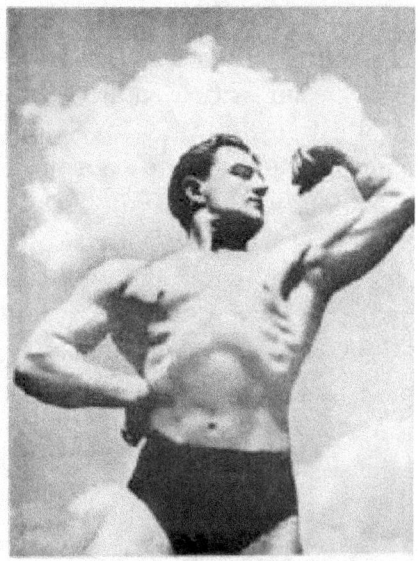

Johnny Terpak, famous middleweight lifter of the York Bar Bell Club

Hercules truly did inspire and does inspire for his massive proportions, his great development, although he is best known for his strength. There were other great figures of the same period—Ajax, Hector, Mars, Atlas, Achilles, the lame God Vulcan and many other heroes of this day so long gone—who glorified the strength and beauty of development of the ancient strong men. These men who have lived throughout the centuries in poetry, prose and sculpture, these great heroes and gods of long ago, are all fine examples of men who possess wonderful, magnificently- developed arms.

The beautiful, well-developed woman, the manly, powerful, symmetrically-constructed man, is always admired in this modern age as in the past. In all of recorded history the ancients enshrined the human body as divine.

The ancient civilizations practically and universally idolized physical beauty and development. And those sculptural masterpieces which have come down to us from ancient days all pronouncedly emphasize beauty of arm development.

The reader is asked to notice that fact the next opportunity he gets to visit an art gallery, especially that section of the gallery devoted to sculptured art. All of these old statues depict models with wonderful arms, for without good arms the human body, male or female, loses much. Well-muscled, larger-than-average arms, with every muscle group so well developed that it imparts size and shape to the arm, always attract favorable attention. During much of the year the coat may be removed and the sleeves rolled up—for comfort first, but the display of well- developed arms thus presented adds much to the personal appearance of their possessor.

Even when clothed, thin, almost muscleless arms can not be hidden completely. And as a man can not go entirely through life wearing his coat there are many times when the development or lack of development of his arms is very evident to all. During the summer weather especially, there are considerable periods when a man will appear without his coat—in rolled-up shirt sleeves, sport shirt, sleeveless jersey, bathing suit or some other form of all-revealing sports costume. Even in formal society, in the most pretentious homes, in the most scrupulously particular walks of society, a man often removes his coat. Many a man has refused an invitation to " please take off your coat and be comfortable " because he knows that his thin, bony, weak-appearing and shapeless arms will show his lack of development and those who see will feel that he lacks manhood. In spite of heat which causes the thermometer to hover around the hundred mark, the undeveloped man will feel more comfortable with his coat on and not wish to have his arms compared with the more powerful limbs of others who are present.

The man of any age, young, middle aged or old, who has good arms will always remove his coat without urging, for he knows that his arms indelibly stamp the minds of others in the group with the fact that he is something of a man, virile, strong and well developed. And he has a right to feel that way. For any man with a well-developed pair of arms should be proud of them and equally proud to show them. It makes no difference what type or kind of humans the people are—men and women, even boys or girls as a class or as individuals—all of them are equally pleased at the sight of a well-developed pair of arms and all of them secretly or openly are envious of the man who possesses powerful, well-developed arms.

Big, well-moulded arms have always been a badge of superior manhood. They always have been and always will be the best method of measuring the strength, development and power of a man, when even partially clothed.

Something or other, some circumstance or other, has drilled into, inculcated into and has impressed into the minds of men and women that big well-rounded arms, with muscles which swell into powerful humps and ridges when flexed, mean that that man possesses strength, virility, power, vigor and health, and that idea is absolutely correct. For large arms do not just grow. They can not be developed by themselves alone. They are the product of all- around physical training, of heavy training or heavy work, of lifting, pulling, carrying. They perpetually show that their possessor is very much of a man.

Some men are naturally broad shouldered, even if not very well developed. They have the underlying bony framework and look reasonably well when clothed. Their clothes partially hide their lack of physical development. But get them into a bathing suit some day and see how they appear. There you will see which is most admired. What man creates favorable attention wherever he may go? Not the man who has shoulders like the hooks in a clothes closet and arms which look like rods with hooks on the ends, but the man who has such a fine development that with fitting pride he could pose for the leading sculptors of the day. No one is filled with pleasure or favorably comments in admiration at the sight of anything ugly, or actually un-beautiful, but beauty, no matter what form it takes, is al-ways provocative of open admiration.

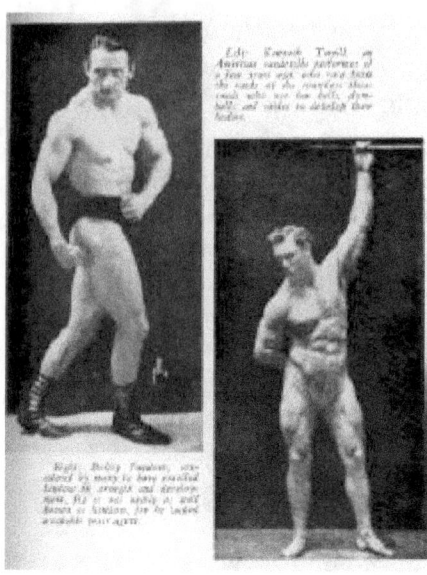

Left: Edward Tuell, an American vaudeville performer of a few years ago, who was known for his fine arms and development. He used bar bells, dumbbells, and cables to develop their bodies.

Right: Bobby Pandour, considered by many to have excelled Sandow in strength and development. He is not using a different position in London, for he looked a notable man at fifty.

It was always thus. It will always be that way. The admiration directed to the well-developed man or woman at the bathing beach today is not a bit different than the heart throbs the maidens of two thousand years ago felt when they saw the fine arms and the accompanying splendid development of the gladiators and the men who raced, played and fought in the arenas of ancient Rome. Artists and sculptors of today seek the best-developed models and big, well-developed arms are always a part of these models just as they were centuries ago.

Herman Goerner, a German who resides in South Africa. He is a great professional lifter and strong man, considered by many to be the strongest man of modern times. His arm and shoulder are well developed at 17 inches.

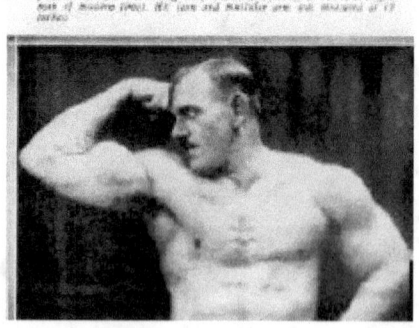

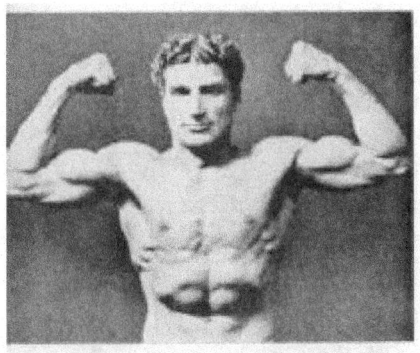

Nicholai Tabutes, to whom the term "Roman anatomical chest" could be applied. He's one of our best developed men of the present and [illegible] in Florence, Italy.

The ancient painters and sculptors who had a real eye for the beauty of the male physique would create statues such as the Farnese Hercules which had arms that frequently remind those who view them of a powerful, wind-swept, gnarled, strong and solid oak tree; while even the most powerful, the best-developed arms of the strength athlete, which are hard as a block of wood when tensed, with muscles standing out like steel cables, are soft as velvet when in repose. The viewer will notice this great difference in statues with tensed muscles such as the Farnese Hercules and in the smooth, rounded, but nevertheless very evidently developed and powerful muscles of other ancient statues. Consider the following sculptural masterpieces. Close examination will disclose the fact that all of them depict wonderful arms. The "Discobulus" or discus thrower, the " Laocoon Group," especially the middle figure of that group, and the seated statue of the ancient god Mars, perpetuate into immortality the real, virile, forceful, powerful armed men who lived in these ancient times.

" Mars Seated " does not just show big arms or wide shoulders. It's a real masterpiece and represents more strikingly and more effectively than many other statues real physical strength, development and beauty. The Apollo Belvedere, long famed as a model of male perfection, is moulded after a figure not so well developed and a bit feminine in appearance. No doubt the original of this statue had the underlying bony framework which resulted in a pleasing appearance, but did not have the development to go with it. Rather than being an athlete, soldier, boatman or workman, he probably was a musician, or poet, at least, of a sort who participated in moderate exercise and athletics only. All of the Apollo Belvedere is strictly feminine with the exception of a better than average pair of shoulders, which as mentioned before can be the result of exceptional skeletal construction.

When looking upon and closely examining " Mare Seated " one is immediately impressed by the intense masculinity it portrays, by the masterly manliness of the entire figure—all the more remarkable because the man who posed for this statue has assumed a perfectly at rest position. The muscles are not tensed in the slightest, but there is force, strength and power radiating from the entire figure. All of the parts of the body blend well together but if you will close your eyes to the remainder of the statue and concentrate entirely on the arms alone, you'll be doubly impressed with the sort of arms a really well-developed and powerful man should have.

Real physical beauty must be harmonious, and there will always be many who admire outstanding development, big muscles, and, I can add again, the biggest of big arms. Harmonious beauty has always been much admired, because the instant any inharmonious element enters into anything, at once any beauty that may be present vanishes. Perfect harmony, balance, all-around development are the true marks of beauty and all of these are found in most of the ancient statues.

The statue known as " Spartacus " portrays most powerful, well-developed arms. The " Hercules" of Tyrian, which represents Hercules carrying away the apples of the Hesperides, also illustrates wonderful arm development.

The statue which reposes in the Louvre, Paris, representing the " Gladiator " is a striking example of masculine beauty and development; it strikingly amplifies the development of the model's arm who posed for it. Michael Angelo's statue of David, made in colossal size (the original of which is in Florence, Italy), again illustrates that the sculptors and painters of every age admired, almost worshipped, power-fully-developed men. Sixteen hundred years passed between the statues of greater antiquity which we first mentioned and this statue of David. But styles don't change in the masculine physique. There have been periods in which the heavy, voluptuous, too well padded feminine figure has been admired; others when the hour glass, tightly-corseted effect was desired; still others when the undeveloped, flat- chested, thin-breasted, round-backed, slouchy type of young women were liked by some; but there has never been a time in world history when the best-developed male physique has not been the style. It will always be thus. For men, and women too, like real men, and real men are the product of exceptional development. As the arms are the most conspicuous part of the masculine physique in the usual modern clothing, it behooves all of us, if we want to look and feel like real men, to spend some time in developing our bodies—especially the arms.

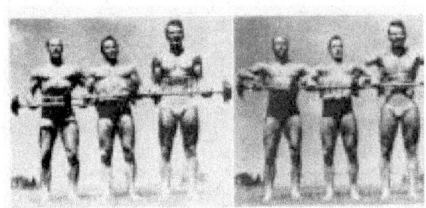

Carol Everidge, Eddie Harrison and Benny Farnham performing the two-hand curl and straight-press(es) motion.

Anatomy of the Arm

IN studying the arm we will start first of all with the bones and levers which make up this part of our bodies. Thus it will be easier to understand the attachment of the muscles, the manner in which the muscles conduct the arm and the way in which the bones of the arm operate and form the various levers. Levers have been known for a great many centuries; in fact, they have been used all through recorded history. The basic idea for their construction has been modeled after parts of the human body. Centuries ago there was no definite knowledge of the formation and operation of the parts of the human body, as dissection was forbidden by law. In the late 15th and early 16th centuries there were many squabbles about the human body—scholars debating whether the body was really as described by Aristotle the ancient anatomist or the more recent dictates of Galen. Both of these opinions or treatises of instruction came as the result of studying animals. It was not until the 16th century that truly authentic information was received, the study and compilation of which was made by Vesalius. Now every medical student makes a close study of human anatomy, the bones and the muscles in particular. A knowledge of the operation, construction and means of development of these parts is helpful to the ambitious body builder.

There is just one bone in the upper arm, the Humerus. In the forearm there are two, the Radius and the Ulna. The Radius is on the thumb side of the arm and is the longer of the two. The construction of the two bones is somewhat similar, both being rather heavy on one end and tapering to a much more slender center of the bone, then enlarging a bit at the opposite end. They are set with the large ends opposite each other, the Radius having its large end as the base for the wrist, the Ulna as the base of the elbow. Medical students always seemed to get a lot of fun out of the fact that the large bone of the arm is the Humerus and to find that it has a great and small tuberosity and a bicipital groove, that it fits into a cavity in the scapula called the glenoid fossa. But intricate descriptions of this sort are unnecessary to the body builder and take up more space than we have at our disposal.

We must consider two bones of the shoulder which have a definite control over the Biceps: the Scapula, commonly known as the shoulder blade, and the Clavicle, which is best known as the collar bone.

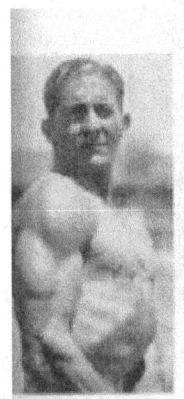 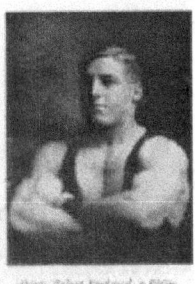

In the body there are three kinds of levers. The bones, muscles and joints form the elaborate system of levers which produce the many diversified forms of motion of which humans are capable. Only a few of the movements are simple, the majority of them including some action of levers.

We have examples of the three forms of levers in the movement of the arms. The first operates with both the power and the fulcrum or attachment at one end and the weight at the other. This movement is best illustrated when the arm doubles up to curl a weight. The second has the point of attachment in the center, the weight at one end and the power at the other. Straightening of the bent arm while pressing a weight represents this second form of lever, and the third with the power at one end, the fulcrum at the other, the weight in the center is best shown by floor dipping. A muscle is said to be inserted at the point of greatest possible movement—to have its origin at the point of least mobility, but there is considerable variation in the attachment of muscles and some of them have their origin and insertion both at the point of greatest movement. The joints of the human body are rather intricate in construction and movement and a clear understanding should be had of their operation. A joint is located where two bones are joined together and it makes possible the movement of these bones. The simplest joint is the hinge, which works not unlike the hinge of a gate and permits but one form of movement, back and forth—the finger and toe joints being examples of the hinge. A great deal more movement is permitted in the action of the wrist and the thumb which comes about because these parts move around two axes with abduction and adduction, flexion and extension all taking place around the one center or joint. The ball and socket joint is represented at the shoulder and hip. These permit pendulum motions front or back, left to right and circumscribing movements round and round. The knee joint permits a twisting action as well as flexion or extension as it is of the spiral type. The base of the skull moves around through the pivot joint which connects it with the axis and atlas at its base.

The elbow joint is a combination of two forms of joints. It more commonly operates as a hinge, but it is capable of twisting motions too. Thus when curling front or back hand it is a hinge, but when rotating as it does in the Zottman, or twisting type of curl, it serves as a screw as well as a hinge. The ankle joint works in a similar manner but directly oposite—the right elbow joint spiraling to the right and just the opposite in the ankle.

The movements of the body are termed flexion which consists in bending one joint such as the elbow or moving one part upon another; extension when extending a limb and straightening the joint; abduction and adduction, the former of which consists in raising one part of the body away from the main part, such as performing the lateral raise, or even the upright rowing motion or the two hands snatch, and adduction consists of bringing the part of the body back to the body again. Circumduction is a circular movement of one of the parts such as the rotation of the shoulders or the arm. Supination is seen in turning the forearm so that the palm is up as in regular curling and refers to turning face up. In the back hand curl, pronation has taken place, the direct opposite to supination which means turning the body face downward or the hand face downward.

Before considering the muscles of the upper and lower arm alone we must give some thought to the muscles of the shoulders and upper torso which control or assist in the operation of the arm to a considerable extent. The Trapezius muscles of the shoulder aid in pulling up the arm, the Deltoid muscles of the shoulder in raising the arm, such as in the lateral raise; the Latissimus Dorsi muscles, the broad band of muscles which impart the shape to the side of the back, pull the arm down. The Subscapular muscle rotates the head of the upper arm bone inward. The muscle which supports the shoulder joint and raises the arm is called the Supraspinatus, while the Infraspinatus rotates the upper arm outward. The Teres Major draws the arm down and back and the Teres Minor rotates the arm outward. These are located on the rear side of the shoulder. The Pectorals pull the arms inward as in operating the Giant Crusher Grip or curling dumbells with stiff arms while lying in the supine position upon boxes or a bench.

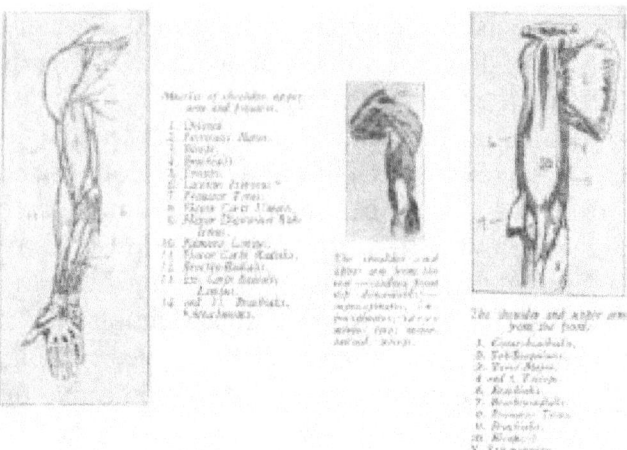

In studying the muscles of the arm, so that we will have a real understanding of its construction, a new vocabulary must be learned. Some of the terms are real jaw breakers such as the Coracobrachialis, the Brachialis Anticus, the Superinator Longus. The most commonly known muscles of the arm are of course the Biceps, which flex the arm, as in chinning or curling a weight to shoulder, and the Triceps of the back of the arm, which plays the major part in straightening the arm.

There are many body builders who believe that the Biceps is the entire upper arm, when as a matter of fact it is only the two headed muscle of the front of the arm. Just this one muscle group can properly be called the Biceps.

In any of the muscle charts shown in this volume you can easily see the relative positions of the Biceps and the Triceps muscles. You will note that the Biceps is hardly one- third of the outer surface of the arms, the Triceps nearly two-thirds. This will give you a better idea of the potentialities of developing large arm size through Triceps building. There is a huge underlying muscle which adds much to the bulk of the arm known as the Brachialis Anticus. It is sandwiched between the Biceps and the

Triceps and only the edges of it appear. But it is responsible for a great deal of the bulk of the well-developed arm. The figure on the upper left of Plate A will give you a clear understanding of the Biceps muscle, so named because of its two heads or points of origin. Both of these heads are attached to the shoulder blades with one of the heads having already passed over the top of the upper arm bone or Humerus. The shorter half of the Biceps has its beginning in what is known as the Caracoid Process of the Scapula and the longer head having its origin at the upper border of the Glenoid cavity of the shoulder blade. Feel your own arm and no doubt you will be able to identify the shorter head of the Biceps as the muscle which goes up under the Deltoid on the inside of the arm. At the lower end, both heads join together in a long flat tendon which is inserted first into the Radius of the forearm, but part of the tendon branches off separately into a part known as the Lacertus Fibrosus or Little Lizard muscle we referred to in another chapter. This tendon joins with the fascia of the forearm muscles and its function is to assist in supination of the arm.

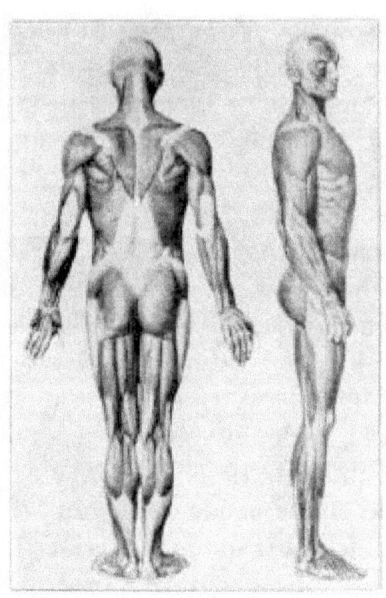

A muscle chart which shows the comparative size of the arm and the muscle groups of the remainder of the body.

Like most of the muscles of the body, the Biceps is not able to work alone, but must always operate in conjunction with other muscles. It has three main purposes: First to curl or bring the hand up to the shoulder, next to turn the foreram so that the palm is up and to assist to some degree in raising the arm out to shoulder height as is done in the crucifix lift, holding weights out from the shoulder palm up. You can feel the greatest strain upon the Biceps group when you perform this movement. The first motion is termed flexion of the elbow, the second, supination of the forearm.

If you refer to Plate B, the figure on the upper right, you will have another view of the muscles of the upper arm. Here the muscles are covered by their fascia with many of the nerves and veins showing. But it does give you a good idea of the relative size of the forearm, upper arm and Deltoid muscles. You will observe that the Deltoid extends about half way down the upper arm to its point of insertion. You can see the advantage in developing the shoulders to build bigger arms. They will not only be bigger but will look even larger as the enlarged Deltoid greatly shortens the appearance of the arm. The figure at the upper left of Plate B was originally intended to show just how the nerves are inserted in the muscles, but it serves our purpose to observe the relative location of the Biceps and the muscles which surround it and work with it.

In the center illustration of Plate B, the little known but highly important (especially for those who strive for size and shapeliness of the upper arm) Brachialis Anticus muscle may be seen. The two heads of the Biceps have been severed near the Deltoid and the Brachialis is exposed. It is a broad flat muscle which lies directly beneath and is practically covered by the Biceps. It may be seen to bulge out when the arm is flexed and in the very well- developed arm its edge can be seen at all times. It has its origin a bit more than half way up the upper arm bone, is fastened to the bone throughout most of its length and then is fastened to the Ulna bone. You will remember that the Biceps is connected to the Radius bone and the fascia of the muscles of the forearm, while the Brachialis Anticus is joined to the other bone of the forearm, thus greatly assisting in the operation of the arm and the power exerted.

Another seldom mentioned muscle of the upper arm which has an important function to perform is the Coraco-brachialis. It assists in raising the arm to the front. It has its origin at the same point as the short head of the Biceps and extends about half way down the Humerus.

The brief discussion this chapter has already contained gives you some idea of the complex construction and operation of the muscles of the arm. We have already described many of the muscles on the front or Biceps side of the arm, the Biceps, the Brachialis Anticus and the Coraco- brachialis. But these muscles would be helpless were it not for the aid they received from the muscles of the forearm group, which are most powerfully involved in all arm movements. We have briefly mentioned the fact that the shoulder or Deltoid muscles extend half way down the arm. The Pectorals or chest muscles have most important attachments in the upper arm, as does tlje Latissimus group of the back; and the muscles of the upper back also have attachments. These muscles with their connections make up a great part of the bulk of the upper arms. More reasons why the men with the best all-around development also possess the most powerful and best-developed, the largest- sized arms.

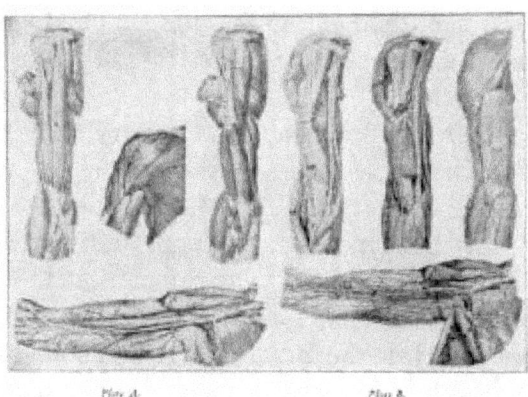

Plate A.   Plate B.

The huge muscle of the posterior part of the arm is called the Triceps, so named because it has three heads, all of which extend into the forearm and on up to the Deltoid. It is the chief function of this powerful group of muscles to straighten the forearm, such as in pressing a weight overhead. It does not push the weight as the uninitiated would at first believe, but straightens the arm by pulling strongly upon the forearm. There is another muscle in the back of the upper arm which is known as the Subanconeus which tenses the ligaments of the upper arm.

There are many students of anatomy who believe that the Biceps is primarily intended to supinate the forearm rather than as a flexor of the elbow. Nevertheless it is easy to determine that the Biceps works best when combining supination and flexion as is always evident in performing a front or regular two hands curl. A close study of the charts which accompany this chapter will help you find other muscles. Checking the chart with the muscles which appear on your own arm when flexed you will find a prominent bulge of muscle on the outside of the forearm which is known as the Brachioradialis. It has its attachment about one-third of the way up the Humerus and its tendon is inserted in the lower end of the Radius. It is primarily intended to be a flexor of the elbow but also performs the functions both of supination and pronation. Whether the hand is turned up or turned down, this muscle has assisted in the movement and serves as a stabilizer to keep the forearm and hand in the position where it can bend or flex the elbow most efficiently. This muscle operates best when the hand is turned so that the palm is toward the body and the thumb uppermost. You will find it much easier to curl a pair of dumbells back hand, with the palms toward the body, than to curl a bar bell back hand, for in this latter position there is some tension or strain upon this powerful muscle.

Examine Plate A again, the left upper figure. Just outside of the muscle we have been describing there is a thin strip of muscle which can be seen even better on the extreme right figure of the same plate. This muscle is known as the Extensor-carpi-radialis-longus, a muscle which helps extend the wrist and aids in the flexion of the elbow.

As you examine the muscles on the outside of the elbow you will see a group of muscles which are the most vulnerable in the human body. I believe that more athletes, baseball players in particular, have injuries to these muscles, strains of more or less severity, than those of any other muscle group of the body. Curling or lifting heavy boxes or other weights, throwing a ball with great effort and terrific speed places an unusual strain upon these muscles, particularly the muscle known as the Superinator. This is a small fleshy muscle directly in the bend of the elbow. It extends up under the Brachialis Anticus and down to the Extensor-carpi-radialis-longus. It is the principal super-inator of the forearm, ably assisting the Biceps in performing that function. It also connects with and assists the action of the Triceps. Again examine closely the right hand figure of Plate B. You will see a cut muscle right at the joint of the forearm. In the illustration at the left of the same chart you can easily trace this muscle as it extends diagonally across the forearm, passing under the Lacertus Fibrosus and the Brachioradialis. Its work is pronation and flexion of the elbow and it is called Pronator Teres.

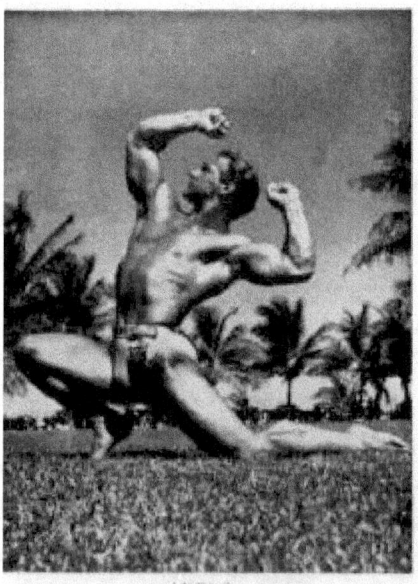

Some body builders endeavor to build their arms almost entirely by chinning and curling. When this is done, only a small portion of the upper arm is brought into intense operation. Dave Mayor, who possesses the largest muscular arms in the world at present, obtained these huge arms, I believe, principally through his fondness for the rowing motion. Of course he is a lifter and does a great deal of snatching and cleaning. In all of these movements the knuckles are up and the Biceps exerts very little effort. It does put forth a little effort in supination, but the actual pulling up of the weight or pulling it to the shoulder as in the back hand curl or the cleaning and snatching motions is done by the Brachialis Amicus. This muscle has been developed to huge size by big Dave Mayor, 265 pounds bodyweight, and accounts for a great deal of the bulk of his 19% inch arms. The two hands chin with the knuckles up will develop the Brachialis Anticus—further proof that the best arms are the product of all around training. The Biceps may offer some slight assistance in performing the rowing motion, but very little; for with the palm turned down to its fullest extent the Biceps is so shortened in relation to associated muscles that it can not perform its •function of flexing the elbow.

Some time spent in closely studying the plates of the arm will be interesting as well as educational. The illustrations show the details of the muscles, the passage of the arteries and veins, the tendons, ligaments, various musclesand the fascia which hold them in place. The left figure on Plate B is so cut that it shows the construction and insertion of the Deltoid. The muscles which extend from the Pectoralis Major are cut and shown in greater detail as well as the muscles which extend from the Latissimus and other parts of the body.

We frequently hear from some man who has trouble with his shoulder joint popping out of place. As a rule this results because the long head of the Biceps muscle is missing, a muscle whose function it is to hold the shoulder joint in place. You can see how this is done as the Biceps tendon passes over the ball of the Humerus as shown on the chart. This tendon serves the usual purpose of a ligament, which works well from every position of the joint and does not restrict the range of arm movement in any direction.

Some persons are minus muscles which are normal in others. It is difficult to determine just how this comes about. Some believe that those who have these extra muscles have acquired them through development during the time of puberty or even earlier, while growth is most rapid. The majority of people do nothing in the line of physical training or exercise, so it would not be surprising if they were minus some muscles. The occupations of many which force them to use their muscles to earn their living could easily account for the development of the extra muscles. In about ten per cent of cases there is an additional or third head of the Biceps which appears midway down the muscle and there are cases of more than three heads. This extra muscle appearing in some individuals is occasionally found in abdominal development, an entire additional row of muscles sometimes being present.

The additional heads of the Biceps of course give their possessors a great amount of muscular advantage. There are variations in the Brachialis Anticus, it being estimated that in about 25 per cent of cases there is a square shaped muscle called the Epitrochlea Anconeus which extends between the Humerus and the Ulna at the elbow. In the people who do not have this muscle there is a strong fibrous band to perform the function of the muscle. A band of course serves as a retainer, but can not exert force. Therefore it's evident that the possessor of the extra muscle has a physical advantage over the man who is without it. The Coracobrachialis is extremely variable in construction in different individuals. It is believed by anatomists that it was originally a three part muscle although it consists of just two parts in the average individual. With some, a separate slip occurs which is known by the large, important sounding name of Coracobrachialis-superior, Coracobrachialis-brevis or by the name of Rotator-humeri,—a lot of big sounding names for so small a muscle, a muscle which is even absent in so many humans. You must have noticed the tremendous names some muscles possess. With few exceptions, the larger the name, the less important the muscle.

There is a great deal more to the anatomy of the bones and muscles of the arm than this chapter has contained; books are filled with the subject. We can not in this small book describe all the parts with great detail. But if any body builders who read this care to take up this study which is a part of the work of the first year medical student, there are good anatomies available, such as Cunningham's, Piersol's or Gray's. What we have offered here should suffice for the usual body builder.

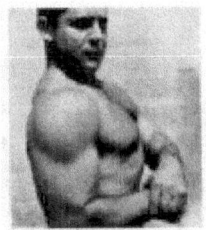

How The Arm Muscles Operate

THE arms are capable of far greater variety of movement than any other part of the body. Although they are assisted in any sport or game, in every vocation, by other parts of the body, they are the connecting link, or the guiding force in nearly every physical operation.

In baseball the hands grasp the bat and impart considerable of the effort in swinging. In rowing they serve as a connecting link between the oar and the powerful back and leg muscles and do much of the finishing of the stroke. In paddling they do a good share of the work; in shot putting, discus, javeline or hammer throwing, they also supply much of the force. In throwing a baseball considerable power comes from the body, but the arms have their work to do as well as being the controlling or guiding force. The arms throw, pitch, toss, lift, carry, push, pull and twist from every conceivable angle. They are so designed that they can exert force in every possible manner and direction. In each of your arms are many millions of muscular fibres which form their muscular bulk and make it possible for them to perform their daily work and to participate in every form of physical activity. Each of these muscular fibres is part of a muscle which is so designed that it can exert energy in the direction in which the mind tells it to pull.

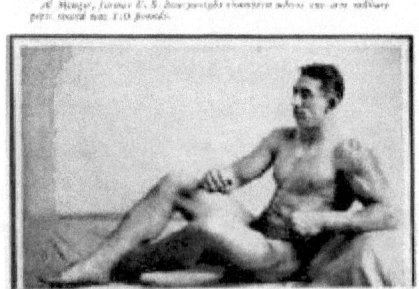

Al Monger, former U. S. low weight champion whose car-arm military press record was 150 pounds.

I wrote pull, for as we will presently see, the muscles never push. Seems odd, doesn't it? One would naturally believe that the arms push while pressing a weight, stretching a pair of cables, dipping on the parallel bars or upon the floor. But the fact is, that a weight is pulled to arm's length as it is apparently pushed overhead. The arm is straightened by the pull of the Triceps against the arm bones.

The shoulder girdle, which to a large measure controls the action of the arms, is most complicated, designed to assist the arms to move from every conceivable angle and to aid them in performing every imaginable movement. Therefore, the construction and function of the shoulder muscles must be considered in relation to the nomenclature and operation of the arms.

Life is movement, it has been said, and movement is solely the result of muscular action. Muscular tissue causes all the movements we experience from birth to the time when we leave the activities of this world. Muscle tissue is a curious substance which exists only in the animal kingdom. It is not fully understood just how the muscular fibres move but we will endeavor to explain what transpires when you wish to throw, pull, lift, or press a weight overhead. In the other form of life on this planet, plants, there is movement of a kind. In fact the great Darwin wrote an entire book about it. The stalks and leaves of plants move and grow toward the sun; frequently they close up at night or during inclement weather. Gasoline or steam generated from some other fuel expands or explodes and pushes against pistons which in turn put gears and wheels into action. Machines push. Our muscles pull.

In some strange manner they have been designed to contract lengthwise more than half their length. The muscle does all of its work by pulling on the things to which it is attached,—the tendons, bones or other muscles. It changes its shape as it contracts to perform its task. It does not get smaller, but expands sideways just as much as it contracts lengthwise. This accounts for the swelling of the Biceps

49

when you " display your muscle." Mechanical engineers have much to learn from the marvelous operating muscular tissue, for nothing else in this wide world operates like muscle.

Development of Muscle

IN the beginning, the later powerful skeletal muscles of the body are little masses of tissue which lie next to the vertebral column. They are arranged like parallel rows of little bricks and when fully grown there are two rows of them, with thirty-five on a side. The muscles of the limbs have their beginning also as little masses of fibres. When a muscle is first formed there are no attachments or tendons. The muscle masses move around as they grow, sometimes wandering to considerable distances from their point or origin. After a time they become adjusted to one another, forming a muscle, which in turn effects a general shape and size, becoming tendinous at the ends. The tendon then will extend the required distance to find its proper attachment. There it becomes attached and settles down, growing fast to a nerve cell so that there is at least one nerve fibre to each muscle. There are about three times as many baby muscles as adult muscles, for only about one-third of them develop. No new fibres are formed after birth and the ones which first go into service must continue to operate for the average seventy years of a human life.

When a muscle becomes bigger and stronger it comes only as a result of exercise. The fibres already present in it increase in size and strength. All muscle fibres can contract automatically. There has been a great deal of study placed back of muscular action, yet the mechanisms of movement are not fully understood. They differ from any processes we know in the physical world and they are very efficient.

Just how do the muscle fibres increase in size? you must be wondering. As we have said, the muscle contracts due to the muscle fibres becoming much broader and shorter in length. This muscular action comes somehow as a result of the direction of the nerve attached to each muscular fibre. Some unknown stimulus of a chemical nature takes place, drawing together the center of the muscle. Just what causes it is not exactly known, but it has been proven that red stripe muscles, when kept alive outside of the body, for some time, regularly, without apparent stimulus, contract over a hundred times a minute. At each contraction a chemical change takes place, some of the materials being changed in nature and waste products formed.

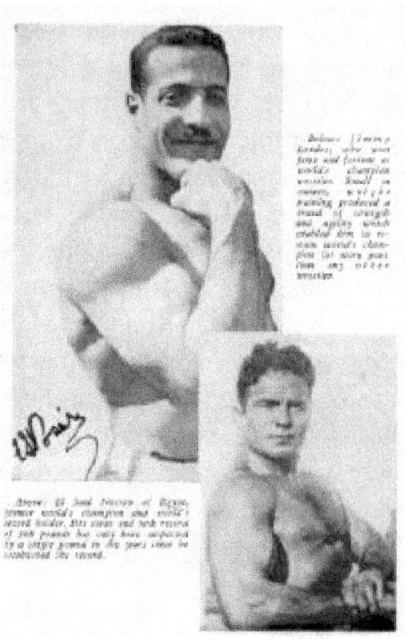

Fatigue in the muscle is felt because an oxygen debt is formed in conjunction with deposits of waste material. It is thought by many anatomists that the glycogen or blood sugar is responsible for the contractile power of the muscle. The glycogen which many believe to be the source of the contractile power of the muscle is apparently formed by the liver. But many believe that the muscles themselves or some other part of the body may have something to do with the function of the glycogen. There is a startling similarity between the changes which take place in the muscle after great exertion and in the muscles after death. The difference of course is the continuance of the bodily processes during life which carry away the waste and replace it with additional elements to supply contractile power.

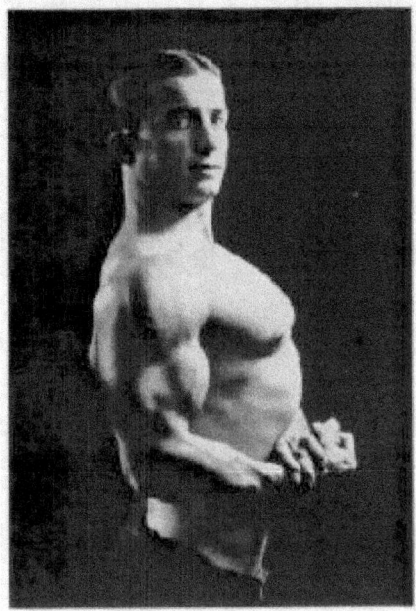

Andrew Pasquale again. Need we tell you that this is one of the finest photos ever shown of the masculine physique?

When a man first takes up the practice of physical training, he will find that he is easily fatigued by a few exercises. But if he should perform a few more movements each day with bar bells or dumbells, in a surprisingly short time his strength and endurance has increased to the point that the resistance first handled, which was quite fatiguing, can now be used with ease. A period of two or three weeks is usually required to break the muscles into the new kind of exercise, to learn the proper positions and to accustom the muscles to the more vigorous contraction.

But as soon as the muscles have become accustomed to the initial poundage and the weights and movements are regularly increased, the strength and health seeker's body will gain in strength and weight, too, in almost direct proportion to the increased weight employed. His chest will become larger, his shoulders much wider; his legs and arms in particular will put on a great deal of muscle. In a short time it's necessary to purchase new shirts, to let trousers out along the seams to fit the ever growing legs.

We have all seen this phenomenon occur. There have been a never-ceasing number of before and after cases pictured in my former books and in every issue of Strength and Health Magazine. Where does all this muscle growth, both in bulk and power, come from? If one of these before cases has started with an arm only eleven inches in circumference £nd that arm increased after three months of specialized training to a girth of fourteen inches and to seventeen inches by the end of the years of training, it means that the muscular bulk of the arm has more than doubled. If the man is mature, the bone will not have grown, so the full increase registered by the tape must be the result of muscular content.

When a man says that his arm has increased from eleven to seventeen inches in girth, first thought would have us believe that it has increased just fifty per cent in size. But if you consider that an arm of eleven inches presents a cross section area of less than eleven inches, while a seventeen inch arm means a cross section of more than twenty- four inches, you will see that the arm has more than doubled in size with this increase of six inches in circumference,— which of course means that nearly every muscular fibre in the upper arm has more than doubled in size.

This great growth has come as a result of exercising the muscles. Vigorous exercise has broken down part of the tissue, and then during the period of rest after exercise, the broken down tissue is replaced and reconstructed by fresh material supplied by the blood, which means that the muscle must be well nourished as well as thoroughly exer- cised in order to grow. We exercise the arm and it grows in size and strength because the exercise promotes the vigor of the digestive and assimilative processes. I briefly mentioned in another chapter that the men who practice all around exercises build the largest arms,—larger arms than the man who endeavors to exercise and build big arms alone. It's granted that any movement of the arm causes some beneficial effect on other muscles of the body, but the exercises which bring all the muscles into action, greatly improving or amplifying the speed of circulation, the volume of respiration, improve digestion, assimilation and elimination, improve the internal processes and amplify the action of the organs and glands which are adjacent to the working muscles, provide the greatest physical improvement and most rapid muscular growth. Bigger arms will be built if these important internal changes, the result of all around training, first take place.

There are several other rules which enter into the building of big arms. The principles of living as advocated by Strength and Health Magazine must be followed. These are simple but highly important. Most important of all is exercise. There will be plenty about that in this volume. Next in value is proper eating. The body must be supplied with the elements it requires to live and function in perfect health. Sufficient rest and relaxation is an essential. That's why the system of training I have always advocated has been so successful. One hard day of training per week in which the ambitious strength and health seeker endeavors to equal or exceed his best efforts of the past; two more days of fairly vigorous training; two easy days for the man who is not employed at work which requires effort from his muscles; and two days weekly of complete rest from unnecessary physical exertion. The rest days bring best results if observed the day before and the day after the more intensive day of training. The maintenance of a tranquil mind is the fourth of the principal essentials. At first thought, it may seem that the mind, an unsettled or troubled mind, should have nothing to do with the development or welfare of the muscles. Scientific experiments have proven that all one needs to do is to become enraged, badly frightened or experience pain and the digestive juices will cease to flow; even the movements of the stomach and the duodenom (the intestines) will cease. Try this on your cat or your dog if you wish to be sure. They will become so enraged with a little teasing that they won't eat. All their digestive and eliminative processes will stop.

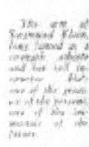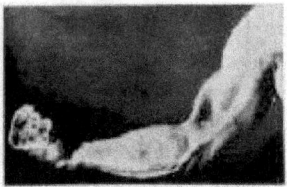

To obtain best results, carefully observe the four essentials of health. It's difficult, well-nigh impossible, to develop muscle, at the same time causing it to become stronger, without having or effecting a thoroughly healthy condition of the internal organs and the vital glands.

Proper nutrition or metabolism is necessary to greatly increase the size and strength of muscles such as the Biceps and the Triceps. In the healthfully functioning human the foodstuffs, after having been consumed, are converted by the digestive juices in such form that they can be absorbed by the blood or lymph. After the oxygen taken from the air has been transferred to the blood, after the blood driven by the heart has been carried through the arteries to all parts of the body, these materials are used for the production of energy first. The oxygen forms a combustion with other properties of the blood and causes the heat and energy on which the movement and well being of the body depend. Most important of all, especially from the body builder's standpoint, is the replacement of broken down cells which takes place through the properties the blood constantly transports.

Metabolism is a little known process. But briefly it consists of preparing the food consumed for assimilation by the blood and then the cells of the body. Just as cutting up logs of wood into small bits which can be fed to a stove supplies heat, metabolism performs a similar function for the human body, supplying both heat and energy.

Carbohydrates, fats and proteins are the materials needed chiefly by the body. There are a few other important substances used in smaller quantities, consisting of minerals and vitamins on which the body depends for health and energy. Briefly the body utilizes six forms of foods: carbohydrates, proteins, fats, water, mineral salt and vitamins. These substances are burned in the body and are utilized to replace waste tissue. At the same time the carbohydrates, proteins and fats yield a certain definite and measurable amount of heat and energy. To build the body, it must be supplied with the foods and minerals it requires, not only in sufficient quantities to maintain it, but with a surplus to depend upon for growth.

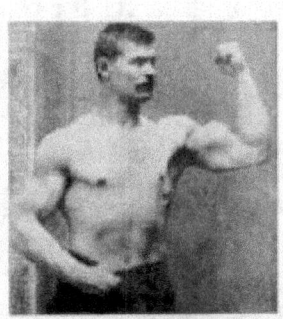

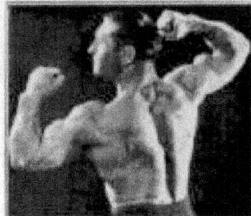

In one of my former books, " How To Be Strong, Healthy and Happy," there is considerable about diet, about the foods needed by the man or woman who wishes to gain or to lose weight. The reader who desires more complete details of the subject of nutrition can obtain the desired information from that big book which covers the subject of health and physical training so much more thoroughly than can a book of this size.

Your muscles, will become larger and stronger as a direct result of the chemical action which takes place within the body. Many people believe that men exercise solely to build muscle. Big muscles are fine. We like them and admire them. But the most important result of modern bar bell and dumbell physical training, or other forms of training with apparatus, is the improved operation of the internal processes. Every organ and gland is benefited which in turn creates the improvement of the muscles. The organs cause the muscles to push, to pull, to lift and to carry. The muscle in itself would be as helpless as the muscles of the dead bull or steer. It's the organs back of the muscles which cause the muscles to grow in size, shape and strength. Therefore, it is evident that only a state of sound health can result in rapid and satisfactory gains in building muscular size and shape of the muscles.

The system of circulation must perform well, carrying the needed elements to the points where they are needed, deep full breathing of good air is an essential to send ample supplies of oxygen to the working muscles, the nervous system must be in such condition that it can properly stimulate the organs and muscles to proper activity, the digestive, assimilative and eliminative systems must first provide proper nutriment for every part of the body and then rid them of poisons which are generated through the action of the parts of the body. Good health is the absence of pain, disease or discomfort of any sort, the proper operation of all the organs and glands. To build big arms, power-ful, symmetrically-developed arms, it's necessary that one conduct one's life so that the maximum of health is enjoyed and the functions of the body operate perfectly.

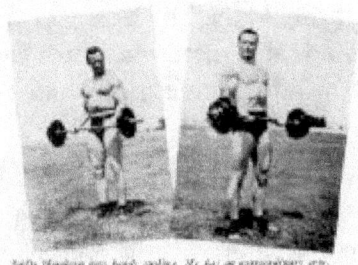

Rudy Thornton two hand curling. He has an extraordinary arm.

Who Has The Biggest Arms?

IN what I have already written you must have noticed that I have been constantly hinting or more than hinting at the fact that the men who never specialize in arm development have the best arms,—the biggest, strongest and best developed,—while many men who do what they believe is specializing in arm development never have a much better than average arm.

This is especially discouraging to some. They work hard and intensively, make curls and chins which run into the thousands and fail to get results commensurate with the effort expended. Then they see some other fellow in their club who has a great arm, one that causes interest and admiration wherever seen, and this fellow does nothing especially to develop his arm. I would say that practically every member of the York Bar Bell Club is in this latter category. Everywhere one looks around our gym are great arms,—not one of them the product of specialization in arm exercises, but all of them the result of all around physical training: lifting first of all; practice of repetition lifting; exercises; most of them have hand balanced, tumbled, worked with cables, dumbells and performed regular body building exercises with bar bells. But there is no special work for the arm. The best shaped Biceps have been acquired as sort of a byproduct of other exercises, not as a result of specialization of any sort.

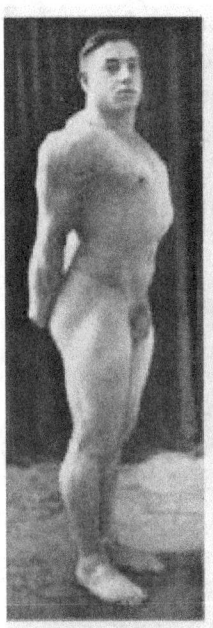
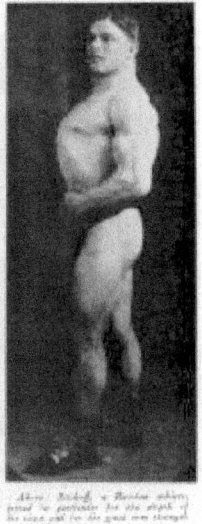

*Above: Bickoff, a Russian athlete,
noted for perfection for the depth of
his chest and for the good arm strength
and development.*

*Left: Charles Rigoulot, of France.
Holder of the world's records in the
one hand snatch, one hand jerk and
the clean and jerk.*

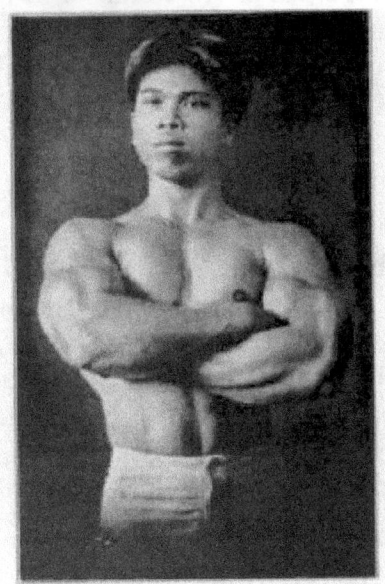

*Young Igakiste, a comparatively small man who possessed one of the
best developed bodies on record.*

The reason for this is probably that the Biceps, being easier
to develop than most parts of the body, does not require so

much work to bring it to maximum development. But it does rely for its development on the function of the internal organs and glands, and these are improved in their operation through all-around physical training; through exercises that not only benefit a single muscle group, but bring all the muscles of the body into action together. This amplifies the operation of the internal organs, which in turn feed the muscles to an extent which permits their rapid growth.

The arms in most movements serve as a connecting link to the huge and powerful back, chest and lower leg muscles. They are operated in many diverse manners in accomplishing their share of handling heavy weights. Instead of performing a great many repetitions with light poundages, the arms of the champion lifter play their part in hoisting great poundages overhead. Think of world's, Olympic and U. S. champion Tony Terlazzo. He weighs 148 pounds and has two hands pressed 255, snatched 250, clean and jerked 335 pounds. The clean and jerk is 40 pounds more than double his bodyweight. How could he help but obtain great development for his arms through building the ability to lift such heavy weights!

The arms benefit not only through the lifting of the weight overhead, but from the reflex action in lowering the weight. Once again I must repeat that all around training is necessary to build the best arms—heavy work, moderate work and some pretty stiff training on other days of the week. The competitive lifters have great arms and there are many men who have developed splendid arms through specialization on exercises such as are contained in this book.

There is hardly a weight lifter who did not at some stage of his weight training career practice every well-known exercise, a great many of which were designed for the development of the arm. It's certainly wise for every young man who wishes to obtain the ultimate in strength and development to spend a lot of time at arm exercises, as well as those for other parts of the body. There will come a time when too much specialization of arm development will not bring the desired results. Then it is better to forego the arm exercises for a time. It's good for all body culturists to have their periods in which they revert to arm developing exercises, then refrain from specialization for a time, for as I have been endeavoring to point out, too much specialization may result in the hard, stringy but not very well developed arm of the endurance lifter or marathon runner.

There has always been a great deal of exaggeration in reporting arm size. This is discouraging at times, when one considers the girth of his own arm in comparison. One good way to prevent much of this would be to carry a tape measure with you and when in the presence of men who are known as the possessors of big arms to suggest that arm measurements be taken. If such practice was the usual order, we would not hear so much of 17 and 18 inch arms.

If you measure another man's arm, be fair, however; help him obtain the largest measurement possible; don't try to make it as small as possible as was done in the case of Wally Zagurski as explained in a chapter of this book. And don't consider that the man is a plain liar, or at least guilty of exaggeration or prevarication, if his arm does not exactly measure to the point where it had been reported. Each man is entitled to the largest possible measurement. I have stated that the arm is biggest in the morning, after some special exercises to pump it to its maximum size and after a certain amount of straightening and contracting the arm to hump the Biceps up as far as possible.

It was five years since I measured my arm. During my special twenty weeks' training demonstration I would measure my arm frequently, usually in the morning, and as

I was anxious to obtain the best arm size I practiced flexing it, humping up the Biceps so that I obtained the 17% measurement I mentioned at that time. I did a great deal of curling. At that time I was at my best at the rowing exercise and particularly the back hand curl. Then there was a period of years during which I did no curls—partly because the regular curl holds no particular advantage for the lifter and somewhat because my Superinator Longus hurt a bit when I attempted curls or chins, or even flexing the arm to the limit.

From the end of 1933 to the beginning of this year I can't remember of my arm being measured. When I dropped in at Richard Villar Kelly's outdoor gymnasium in Havana in January, 1938, immediately he brought out the tape measure. I had no idea what my arm was at that time. He measured my forearm at 14 and the upper arm at 17. The upper arm measurement was less than I had mentioned or claimed in the past, yet it represented a really bigger arm. First, pumping up the arms would result in as much as a half inch gain. Next, the practice of flexing the arm to the limit would develop the ability to hump the Biceps up to a greater extent and thus obtain a larger measurement. I had done no curling for years, so my Biceps was not as good as it was. In spite of a smaller measurement than I had claimed, I am sure that had I ever measured my arm straight five years ago and now, my arms are bigger. Within the last few weeks I have found myself able to perform front curls for the first time in years without some slight pain, and should get my arm size up to a greater measurement than ever before in my life. This would be natural, for I am older, should have more adipose tissue, especially as I weigh more, I can lift much more weight, am definitely stronger. While in Cuba due to the heat my fondness for fruit juices which could be had in copious quanities, I am sure I drank gallons of fresh fruit juice, and the fact, too, that I wanted my waist to be as slender as possible for the exhibitions and the swimming and fun at the beach, I had reduced more than ten pounds in bodyweight. Ten pounds lost come from all parts of the body, even the arms and legs. When a man is down in weight, all his measurements are reduced too.

Take all sorts of facts such as these into consideration when you measure a man's arm: The time of day, whether the measurement is taken cold or after exercise, whether he weighs the same as at the time of claiming a certain measurement. I believe if he comes within a half inch of the claimed measurement that you can give him the benefit of the doubt and believe that you have found the honest man that Diogenes, the ancient Greek philosopher, spent so many years of his life in search of.

Big arms are scarce. Arms which may look huge are often much smaller in actual measured girth than you would expect. And some body builders hear so much of the advertised measurements of others that they can almost be pardoned for stretching a bit in their own cases to keep up with the other fellow. Some men add an inch or two, and this isn't enough to keep up with the man who has apparently multiplied to obtain his own advertised measurement. Probably that's the way Sandow's arm grew from the inches at which Dr. Sargent measured it to the 19 inch size which he or his ghost writers reported. He was believed by many to be the strongest man in the world; actually there were many bigger men who were stronger and of course weighing as they did a hundred pounds or more than Sandow would have bigger measurements. The majority believed that arm size denoted the strongest man, so Sandow just had to try to keep pace and add to the size of his arm.

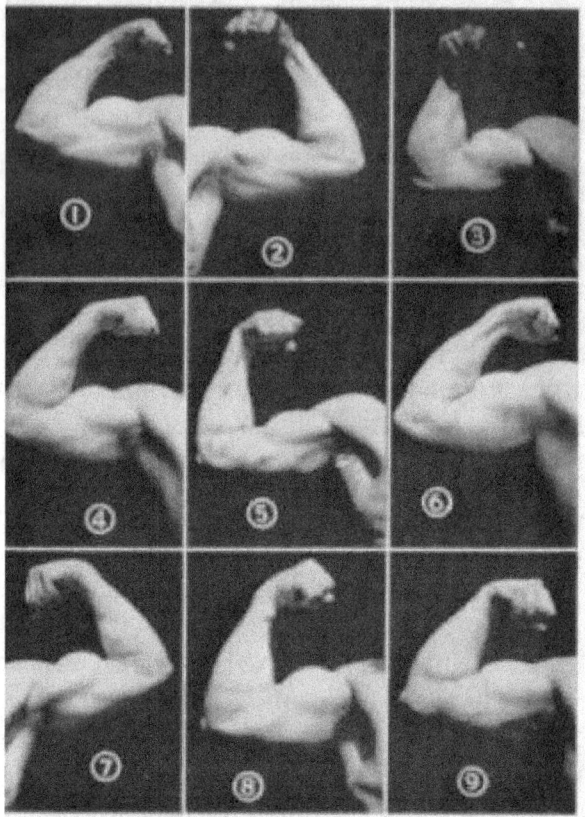

Arms of some of the greatest strength athletes of the present. 1. Eddie Harrison. 2. Tony Terlazzo. 3. John Grimek. 4. Weldon Bullock. 5. Gordon Venables. 6. Mike Dietz. 7. Johnny Terpak. 8. Bob Mitchell. 9. Dave Mayor.

If you've seen pictures of Sandow's arm, you will agree that it is about as fine, well developed, shapely and large for the size of the man as it could be. He weighed, according to Dr. Sargent's report, 180 pounds. A 16 1/2 inch arm at that bodyweight comes very close to being the limit in arm size which could be expected, I believe.

There has been a great deal of mystery about John Grimek's measurements. He told me that he does not believe in measurements, and will write an article very shortly to prove his contention. Proportions, shapeliness and strength he considers of much greater importance. He knows too that it is difficult for the man with honest measurements to compare even remotely with the man who has stretched his measurements. In obtaining measurements of the York Bar Bell lifters, I did not intend to insist that he give me his dimensions owing to his belief that measurements are not of value, but he came into the office where we were obtaining the measurements of others and volunteered to have his arm measurements taken. There have been many thousands of requests to tell of Grimek's measurements, but I doubt if ever before have they been published.

I believe that John Grimek has the most magnificent arms of any of the strong men, athletes or lifters of history. He weighs less than big Steve Stanko, and has almost identical measurements. He is considerably shorter than Steve, perhaps four inches, so the same arm girth looks truly tremendous on John Grimek, for Steve's huge arm looks' almost like someone's leg. I mentioned elsewhere in this book that Grimek had arms of 18V2 inches when he weighed his highest upon the return from the Olympics in 1936. I said that he had an 18 inch arm at his normal bodyweight of just over 190. And the tape bore out my estimates very closely.

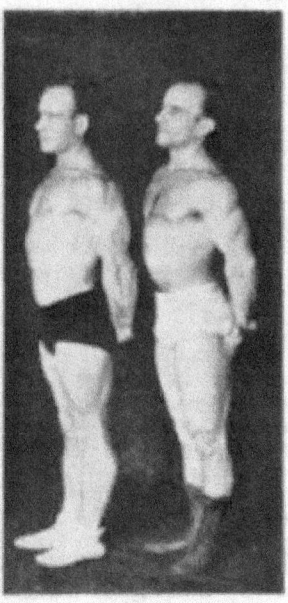

When Grimek holds his arm straight, you would be astonished at the tremendous curve of the Triceps, so his arm measures the same as Steve's straight—i6Vs inches. He has the ability to hump his Biceps up higher than Steve's, so in position No. i his arm is 17 1/2 inches. In positions No. 2 and No. 3, he has the same measurements—He has a little larger forearm than Stanko, 14 3/4 straight and 16 inches flexed. Although there are pictures of Grimek's arms in this book, you will never appreciate the truly marvelous arms he has developed until you actually see them. I am sure that I am not exaggerating when I say that never before or now has there been another pair of arms just like Grimek's. And if he would permit his body- weight to go up, as he can so easily, he would no doubt reach the 20 inch class of arms which so few have attained. John Grimek is more interested in proportions, in shapeliness and strength, than just big measurements, so he controls his weight and physique at a point which he believes is best suited for his bony framework.

If you were to measure many arms which are claimed to be 16 inches, you'd be surprised to learn that many of them, which really look to be 16 inches, are but 15 or even as low at 14%. Very few heavyweights have more than a 16 inch arm. We have had some of them in York— Mayor, Grimek, Stanko, and Bullock—whose arm size has been mentioned a number of times. There have been a few men in this country who had actual 18 inch arms. I have seen a number of them measured, but all of these men carried considerable excess weight and much adipose tissue on the arms. The late John Mallo, heavyweight champion of 1933 was one of a group who lifted in that year's championships who had 18 inch arms. John Curtis Hise of Homer, Illinois, was another and George Mansor, who shortly afterward went into professional wrestling, was another huge youngster, 255 pounds in bodyweight, who had greater than 18 inch arms. Dave Mayor first attained an 18 inch arm in 1936, Then he was not nearly as heavy as later in his career and his arms were quite muscular and thin skinned. As his arms grew they lost considerable of the shapeliness and the muscular definition they had at first, I thought.

Weldon Bullock, when he weighed 240, had a fine arm which was measured at 18 inches. Gregory George of St. Louis, a heavyweight sensation of this year, weight 257, height less than 6 feet, has 18 inch arms and although I have never had the opportunity to measure them I am sure that A1 Senecal of Rhode Island has at least 18 inch arms. But all of the men I have enumerated are not only very big men, far over 200 pounds, usually 230, 240, 250 or even more, but they are all very strong too. All have clean and jerked well over 300 pounds; most of them have made lifting totals of 800 or more, and to make 800, lifts such as 240 press, 250 snatch, 310 clean and jerk are required. There are not more than ten men whose arms I know to be or to have been more than 18 inches.

Eighteen inch arms are quite rare and 17 inch arms are nearly as rare. They are not found on any men except those of good size and with phenomenally developed arms. A 17 inch arm on a man who weighed 180 pounds would be most extraordinary. As we have said, Sandow at 180 had a 16V2 inch arm (that is average girth); his left arm was measured at 16.1, the right at 16.9. The report of Dr. Sargent does not indicate whether Sandow pumped up his muscles before these measurements were taken. He did perform a great many lifts and strength tests, but the report of 1892, when Sandow was 26 and these measurements were taken, does not tell us whether the tape was used prior to the strength and agility tests or afterwards. Probably specialization would have resulted in a 17 inch arm for a man of Sandow's weight of 180, who was as magnificently muscled as Sandow.

Of present day athletes, Wally Zagurski has one of the finest arms in proportion to bodyweight. His arm is now 17 inches, his weight approximately that of Sandow. But to make up this 180 pounds, he has a much better upper body development than lower limbs in spite of the fact that they too are powerful and well developed. It would seem that Wally has reached a very high degree of arm development in proportion to bodyweight.

John Davis, as every lifter or reader of Strength and Health Magazine knows, is most extraordinary. He's U. S. and world's champion, world's record holder, can chin repeatedly with one hand, holding weights in his hand. He pressed 290 pounds when he himself weighed 190. Yet his arm is just i6V2 inches. Quality of muscle and proportions in his case truly mean more than size.

While there are many other good arms among the champion lifters of the York Bar Bell Club, I believe that none can surpass Tony Terlazzo's arm in size and shapeliness for his bodyweight. It's about as huge an arm as a man of 148 pounds could hope to attain. Tony's measurements are as follows: Forearm straight, 12%; flexed 14; upper arm No. 1 position, 15; 15% No. 2 position; and i6Vs No. 3 position. These are truly Herculean measurements. And we must consider the fact that Tony holds all the United States lifting records in the 148 pound class, most of them in the featherweight class, and holds world's records in both of these classes. He's the greatest lifter, in proportion to bodyweight, the world has ever seen. He believes in exercise too and has practiced every one of the 101 dumbell exercises and a few besides, and every one of the cable, crusher, and lifting exercises, as well as rope climbing and balancing. His arm is a product of all around training, repetitions, more moderate poundages and very heavy weights.

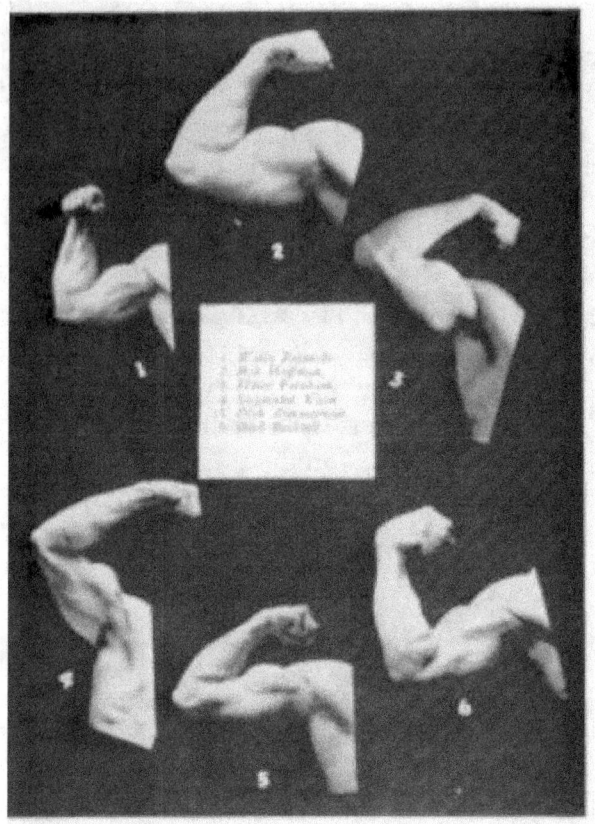

Nine arms of the world's best weight lifters—members of the York bar bell club.

Eddie Harrison is another who has a truly fine arm. He is second only to Terlazzo in lifting ability, having been runner up in the 148 pound senior national championships in 1938 and 1939. He was formerly junior national champion and champion of North America. He has power as evidenced by a 235 snatch and a 300 pound clean, more than double his body weight. His arm is 14 1/2 in No. 1 position, 15 1/2 in No. 2, and 16 inches in No. 3. Eddie has one of the finest arms I have ever seen, growing more impressive in appearance with each passing week of training. In addition to lifting and all around weight training, he is a fine hand balancer, being the understander in an act with

Val de Genaro, a man of his own weight. Usually the top mounter weighs a great deal less than the understander, but Eddie handles his own weight in every phase of the act. His forearm straight is 12 1/2, flexed 14.

Johnny Terpak is a famous lifter, national champion year after year, holds all the U.S. records in his class; he won the world's championship at Paris. He's light in his class, 160 in the 165 division; not nearly as powerful appearing as one would expect when considering his best lifts of 250 press, 260 snatch and 330 clean and jerk, lifts which total 840. He has powerful arms, but somewhat different in shape from the average outstanding strength athlete. While many of the best developed men have Biceps which bunch up close to the Deltoid, and a Triceps which curves evenly on the under side of the arm, so that it is not possible to obtain the greatest Biceps measurement in relation to the Triceps without slanting the tape, Johnny has a Triceps which is thickest toward the shoulder. Any man who has the power to press 250 has real Triceps strength, but there was a slight difference in construction in Johnny's arm as compared to any other. His measurements are: Straight upper arm, 13 3/4; No. 1 position, 15; No. 2, 15 1/2; No. 3, 15. From these figures you can see that Terpak has a powerful arm, but lacks the swelling Biceps of Terlazzo's arm. Nevertheless, Johnny possesses power to a superlative degree as his lifts, in proportion to bodyweight, rank among the first three or four in the world. His forearm straight is 12 1/2, flexed 13 3/4.

I measured the arm of a very slender young man who happened to be in the office at the time of measuring these other arms. His arm straight was 9% inches; No. 1 position, 10%; No. 2, 10%; No. 3, 11%; his forearm straight, flexed, 11 Vie- In the case of this slender arm, which happened to be rather well developed, the largest point of the forearm was about two inches below the elbow as in the case of the bigger arm, and you'll note that the size of the arm had the same relation of measurements as the bigger arms in 1, 2 and 3 positions. This man is very light boned, of average height, but low in bodyweight. He is interested in bar bell work, and it will be interesting to watch his progress from his 11 inch arm to one of 15 to 17 which he will acquire with persistence.

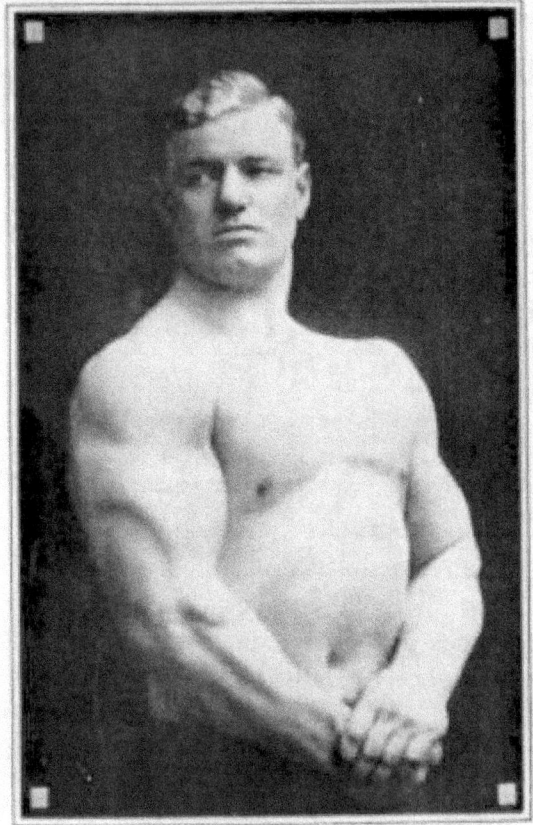

Joe Nordquest. Although handicapped through the loss of a lower limb as a lad, he developed the great physique shown here and established records in hand pressing and floor pressing.

Mike Dietz measured as follows: 13 3/4 straight upper arm; No. 1 position, 15 3/4 inches; No. 2, 16 1/4,; No. 3, 16 3/4; forearm 13 3/4 straight; flexed 14 3/4. Mike is a very powerful young man, weighs about 180 pounds, has good measurements considering that his work is accounting, which permits very little training time. Val de Genaro is a good lifter, one of the best 148 pound men in the country. He's a better acrobat and performs some feats which rank him among the first flight of acrobatic performers. His measurements were as follows: Upper arm straight, 14% inches; flexed, 14% inches. This comes about because he has a very unusual Triceps development— partially the result of hand balancing, running about on his hands, climbing and descending steps in the hand stand position, balancing on his fingers, and finally two thumbs and one finger, three points in all. He's also a very strong man, a good jerker, 290 being his record, but 265 is his best clean. Lack of Biceps development no doubt has much to do with this ordinary cleaning ability in proportion to his other lifts. He's the bent press champion of America in the 148 pound class. And the bent press is a very good Triceps developer. His forearm straight is 12 inches, flexed 13. Once again this is the result of hand balancing and finger balancing to a considerable degree. He has an unusual relation between the forearm straight and flexed.

Lou Schell, one of the best featherweights in the country, was measured next. He's tall for his weight, quite powerful, snatches 170, cleans and jerks 235, presses 170 with very moderate training. His upper arm straight is 12; No. 1 position, 13; No. 2, 14; No. 3, 14 3/4. He performs a one-arm dead lift with 350 pounds and has unusual strength for the size of his arms.

Dick Bachtell, another featherweight, but not nearly so tall, a man who has a magnificent arm in proportion to his weight, one of the world's best, measured 14 in No. 1 position; No. 2, 14 3/4; No. 3, 14 3/4,—a very good arm for a man of his size. Dick is five feet two inches tall and has most unusual calf and arm development.

These measurements should give you a very good idea of the proportion of upper arm you should have for your bodyweight, when developed to near its limit. It would not be possible to build an arm that exceeds to any great degree the arm measurements I have given you, for these men are among the world's best strength athletes, the best all-around performers. They have followed a training system which develops the muscles from every angle and has built power, muscular size and splendid proportions. If you can obtain an arm such as any of the men mentioned have built, providing you are the same height and weight, you'll have a truly impressive pair of arms, which will stamp you as one of the best wherever you may go.

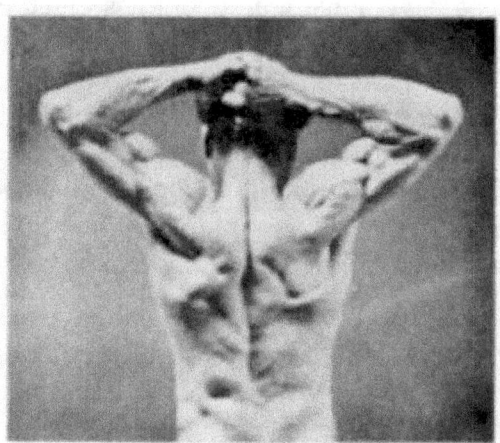

Michael Salvant again. Seldom can the Brachialis Anticus, the deep lying muscle between the Biceps and the Triceps, be seen as clearly as in this photo.

The Finest Upper Arm Development

IN this book you will see a great many finely-developed arms. There is some slight difference in shape between these arms. Most of them have a rounded or ball like Biceps muscle which completely fills the space between Deltoid and forearm. Some arms are apparently more developed than others, having a shorter, higher hump of muscle. This is the result of having attained the limit in development, or a physical characteristic of the individual. You must constantly watch and measure the upper arm to see if you continue to progress. If the tape shows a satisfactory increase, then you are on the right track and can continue the training methods which are bringing good results.

But if you fail to gain after a considerable period of upper arm specialization, you should moderate your efforts a bit—practice no special arm exercises for a time, just take them as they come in one of the regular courses. Then after a period of rest you should be able to go forward again. The individual himself is the only one who can decide just how much of special arm work he can stand.

There has been considerable talk and writing in the past by those who feel the green eyed monster of jealousy, when they compare their own physical self with the bodies of advanced weight men; about their preference for long, smooth, lithe, athletic muscles. They would not want the gnarly, lumpy muscles of a weight lifter. To answer these gentlemen: There is no great range of difference in the length of the muscles. They are determined by the length of each man's bones and from the point of attachment they can not be lengthened or shortened. But they can be thickened and enlarged a great deal which in conjunction with a much better developed Deltoid muscle, the attachment of which extends half way down the Humerus bone, and a very well developed forearm which extends well up the arm, will make the upper arm appear shorter.

Undeveloped men have a Biceps which looks about as big as an oyster or a peanut. They may blame this on some peculiarity of their construction. But the only possible peculiarity that may be present is their lack of development. They can usually hump this little muscle up to a fair degree. There is a very considerable interval between the end of this muscle when flexed and the forearm. I have seen arms in which the lump of the Biceps when flexed is tight against the Deltoids. The possessors of such arms have marveled at the swelling, space-filling volume of the really well-developed arm.

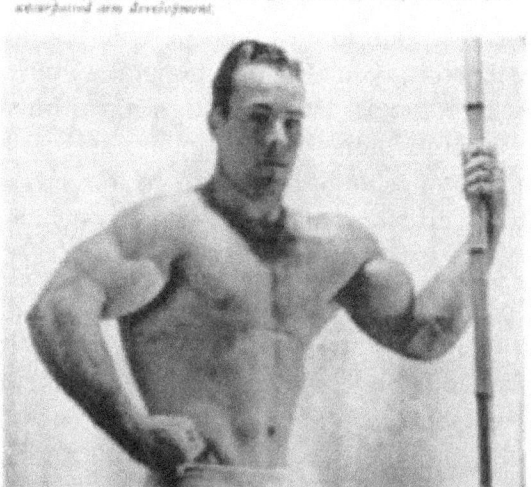

Cliff Byers—A little known strength athlete of today who has won exceptional arm development.

All the man with this type of development requires is greater bulk, more development. And it's difficult to build the desired development without increasing the entire body- weight. So if you are one who follows some unnatural system of dieting, if you are a vegetarian, or practice any other rules which rob the body of all the materials, fats, carbohydrates, proteins, minerals and vitamins it requires, change your eating program so that you can put on some of the weight you need. Exercise the entire body. Build your strength and endurance to the point where you can handle really heavy poundages in all the exercises. Improve all the processes of the body, the internal works, organs and glands as well as the exterior muscles. And this is the result of following the rules of health, particularly of exercising.

People die when the operation of one of the organs of the body fails. Well built, apparently healthy and strong men die every day through heart failure. If the failure of one organ causes death, it's natural that a faulty action or impairment of one of the organs would retard the process of developing, increasing the weight and size of the arms, as well as other muscles. First take inventory of yourself, see what omissions or commissions may be responsible for your failure to gain. Then change your living habits to an extent that you can continue to progress and build a physique which ranks with the best in the land.

A Biceps or Triceps which can be flexed into a lump almost as hard as a piece of wood may be the result of great development and it may be a characteristic of the particular individual. It may be the result of too finely drawn a condition in which the muscles almost try to push their way through the skin. Such a condition is not to be desired. Far better that there be a certain amount of adipose tissue, or thin layer of fat, which provides a reserve, something for the muscles to work upon when they need it. Adipose tissue may prevent some of the separation of muscles from being so evident, but it will provide the much desired bulk, and with well developed muscles underneath they can still provide a most interesting display.

Some men have flesh which is naturally hard. You must, at times in your life, have seen salesmen, professional men or teachers who perform no manual labor, who could display an arm with humps and bumps, veins and sinews and brag about their development with little or no exercise. They are usually of the thin type. Then you have seen rather corpulent men who had huge arms, but there was no evidence of muscle there. Yet these men were terrifically strong and able to lift great weights. Men like Louis Cyr, Horace Barre, Cyclops Bienkowski, Anzan, and others of their type had huge, smooth, but terrifically strong arms.

You should strive to hit the happy medium between these arms and the too thin, stringy, hard and yet undeveloped arms which stretch the tape to a full eleven or twelve inches. A smooth arm can be lack of condition, lack of training. But more than likely it is the type of the man to have such an arm. During my entire athletic career, from a body weight of around 160, I have never had muscles which stood out in bold relief. They were always quite smooth in development and as they served me especially well in many branches of athletics I should not have complained. Nevertheless, like so many others I was something of a muscle worshipper. I thought that perhaps the smoothness of development of my own arms was the result of practicing every possible exercise and following every branch of athletics. I thought that perhaps concentration on one line of training for some months would bring out the particular muscles involved. I was always ambitious to row for the famous Vesper Boat Club in Philadelphia and one year I arranged my business so that I could do that. After six months of intensive rowing, mixed with a little specialization on Biceps work, I weighed just 177 pounds and looked exactly the same in development as when I started the rowing season weighing somewhat more. The smoother type of arms will usually perform best for their owner. They can be " hard as a rock " or just firm to the touch depending upon the type of flesh of the individual.

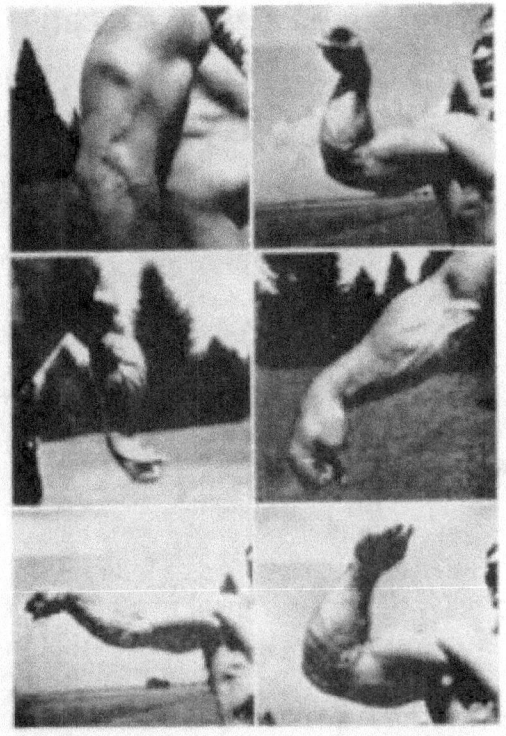

John Grimek's arm from various angles. Too bad that you can't actually see his magnificent arms. Part is lost when the photo is taken, when the engraving is made and in printing. There is still plenty left. But no picture can do justice to a physique such as this man, whose photos appear in this book, posses.

The star lifter's arms in repose, while well muscled and shapely, are soft to the touch. It's their power in flexing these muscles which brings them to the very hard and knotty appearance that those who don't have them and feel the green eyed monster of jealousy decry against.

Follow the rules of health, continue to train as the tape and your own feelings decree and you are sure to obtain the desired results in the end.

Impressive Feats of Strength

You have developed your arms and your grip to a considerable extent, there are many impressive feats you can perform. Lifting humans in diverse ways is one of the best ways to demonstrate your strength. It's difficult for a witness to realize that bar bells are so heavy when you lift them and that just the addition of a " few of those little washers " on the end of the bar is the difference between an ordinary lift and a record. You can allay the onlookers' suspicion by urging them to lift the weight just off the floor which you hoist to arm's length overhead. People know that humans are heavy and when they see you lift them to arm's length, with one hand or two, they are sure that you are quite strong.

A favorite feat of the old time strong men in particular was to resist the pull of a score of men, two horses or even two autos in the early days of the now familiar mechanical contrivance which serves us so well. The common way of performing this feat was to clasp the hands in front of the chest, fasten straps to the arms and then a long rope to which a number of men would apply their force. The chief difficulty with this feat is to get both groups of men to pull simultaneously. If they don't, it's more than difficult for the strong man to retain his equilibrium first of all and to withstand their pull second of all. The great Appollon of France had his Pectoral muscles torn withstanding the pull of two autos. Some autos even in those days had more than fifty horse power and it is not to be expected that human flesh could withstand such a pull. Many strong men had a device made which they could grip, making possible the resistance of a great deal more weight. Broad straps should be employed so that the muscles will not become bruised.

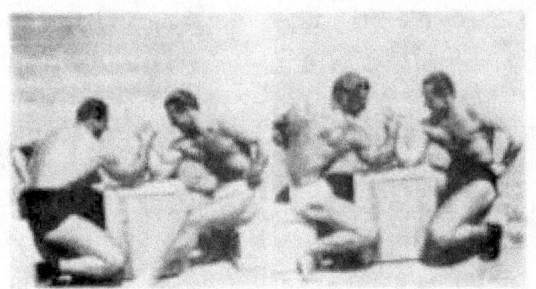
Who do you think will win? Steinke or Grimek.

Wrist wrestling is a favorite with strong men everywhere. Proficiency at wrist wrestling is more often the result of skill and practice than just power in the beginning. Two men face each other upon opposite sides of a small table or narrow counter. Hands are offered to each other, elbows rest on the table, palms together. At a signal, each tries to force the other's hand to the table. Some men start with a pull toward them which gets the other man off- balance and places him in such a position that he can not resist and is an easy victim. A sudden start will often win. But if both men play fair, and exert their strength fairly and evenly, the strongest man should win. There is a form of hand wrestling which requires considerable strength. Two men stand facing each other so that their toes touch. Their hands are clasped and the idea of the stunt is to pull the other man in such a way that he will lose his balance and step forward or back or get off-balance to the point that some part of his body other than the soles of his feet will touch the floor.

Try this one. Place the palm of your hand on top of and to the opposite side of your head. Extend your elbow. Now ask anyone to attempt to dislodge your hand. If you are strong, the other fellow won't be able to budge it.

Stand with your back flat to the wall. Place your hands on hips, elbows front, and defy anyone to push your elbows back against the wall.

You can learn to lift other persons of most any size principally with arm strength and then prevent them from lifting you. When you lift the other fellow, hold your elbows against the hips. Curl him or her from the floor much as you would perform a two hand curl with a bar bell. But when they go to lift you, hold your hands against their arms so that the arm has a bend of greater than a right angle. With your thumb, exert pressure at the side of the Biceps. They will find themselves unable to move you and the usual onlooker will think you are so much stronger.

One hand dipping is always impressive. You can learn this by resting most of the weight on the hand which you wish to dip with. In the beginning, provide a bit of help with the other hand. Gradually diminish this assistance until you are able to perform not one but many one hand dips. This was a favorite exercise with Dave Mayor early in his lifting career. Big as he was he could perform twenty consecutive dips and certainly it was a contributing factor in building that huge arm of his.

Most advanced strength athletes can chin with one hand. Many of them can chin with a weight held in the other hand. I remember reading years ago that no one could chin with one hand without a bit of cheating—starting with a bent arm, or twisting in such a manner that the Latissimus does most of the work. But there's hardly a man in the York Bar Bell gym, for instance, who can not perform it correctly and fairly. The smaller men do it with absurd ease, although this article of long ago said that they did not believe any man could chin fairly with one hand, certainly no one but the smallest. Johnny Davis, world's light-heavy champion, weighing 190 pounds, has chinned repeatedly with a 25 pound dumbell in the other hand. That's a weight of 215 pounds. And Steve Stanko, weight 220, can chin several times.

Paul Holloway of York chins with one finger. This is especially commendable because he is a powerfully developed young man, having very heavy legs. The usual gymnast who learns to chin with one hand will have light legs, but all of these lifters have most powerful lower limbs.

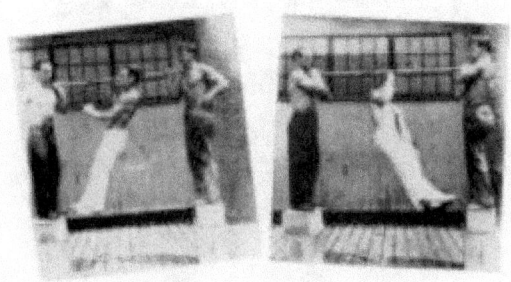

Paul Holloway, chinning with one finger.

Constant practice of lifting motions and actual lifting and preliminary training with curling and rowing, have built the power to perform a one hand chin for these men of the York Bar Bell Club and for so many others. To learn to chin with one hand: Reach the stage of ability to chin fifteen or twenty times with both hands. Then after pulling yourself up with two, let yourself down, suspending all or part of the weight of the body with one hand. Later, in pulling up, do most of the work with one hand, just a bit of aid from the other. Gradually diminish the effort of the non-chinning hand until you can perform a chin with one hand. In the beginning, you can grasp the chinning wrist with the other hand and aid in that manner. Other feats you can learn with arm and hand strength will be included in the chapter on developing the hand and the grip.

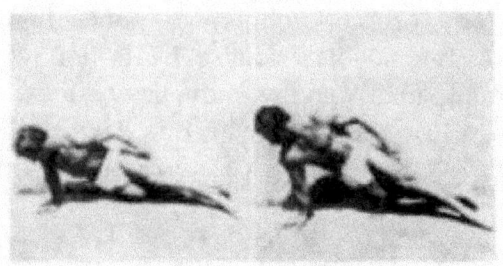

Grimek dipping with one hand.

Why Don't I Have Bigger Arms?

I AM in contact with many thousands of ambitious body builders. They visit me here at York and I see them at lifting and strength shows over much of our broad land. The most common questions they ask are, " How can I gain weight? How can I increase my measurements? " My answer is always the same. There are no secrets in obtaining either of these ends. Just follow the advice I have offered in my articles in Strength and Health Magazine, or in my various books and you should obtain satisfactory results.

In the chapter of this book, " Development of Muscle," I endeavored to illustrate the necessity in gaining weight and strength by following the rules which consist of healthful living. The younger or immature man, the underweight man or woman of any age, who wishes to gain weight, must follow the rules offered, consume plenty of foods which aid in weight gaining and exercise intelligently.

Some men gain more rapidly than others. I often liken their cases to a fertile, unused field of good soil. Plow, plant, cultivate. Every nation, every race, every color, has its strong armed men and love for strong crop results. The ground is fertile and ready for the seed. But there are run-down, impoverished farms, where year after year there have been planting and cultivation without feeding the land with animal or commercial fertilizers. The ground reaches the point where it will not produce even a fair crop until years of careful cultivation and fertilization have taken place. Some individuals are in the same position. Either through heredity, or the life they have lived, they are not in a state of health which will permit the rapid gains of the former case I described. They must spend a much longer period of feeding and cultivating the muscles. They may suffer from stomach trouble, from constipation or other ills or physical irregularities. Regular training as we related before will improve the action of all the organs and glands. First improve all the functions, and in time the desired gains will be made.

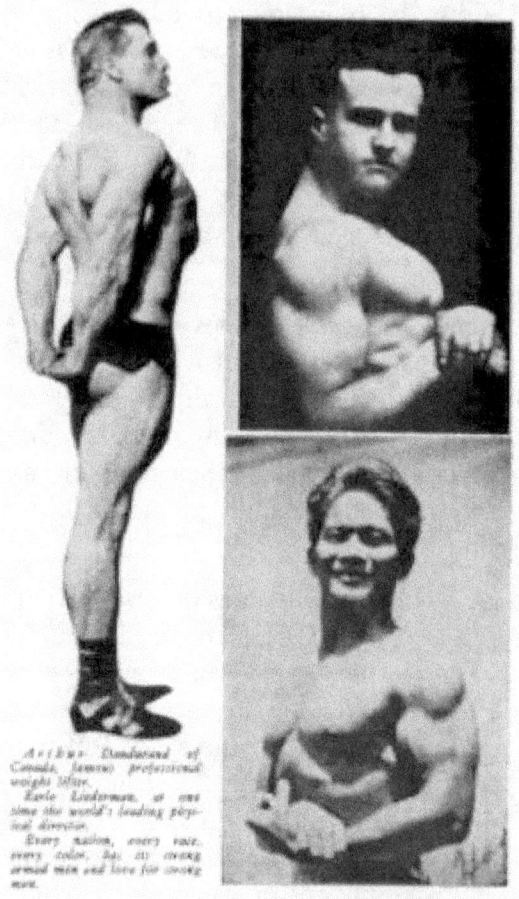

It requires a longer period for some men, much more effort than for the fortunate fellow who either through heredity or the life he has led has a body ready to respond immediately and in a large way to physical training. I try to analyze the particular conditions which are brought to my attention. I ask them what sort of a cook they have at home, the sort of meals served, the variety of foods they regularly eat. Too many people get in eating ruts, consuming day after day and year after year the stereotyped American meal of meat, any kind, too often fried, pickled or dried, potatoes, white bread and coffee. Not nearly enough variety. The body can not obtain from such rations all the fats, proteins, carbohydrates, minerals and vitamins it requires. It will be lacking in strength and resistance to disease.

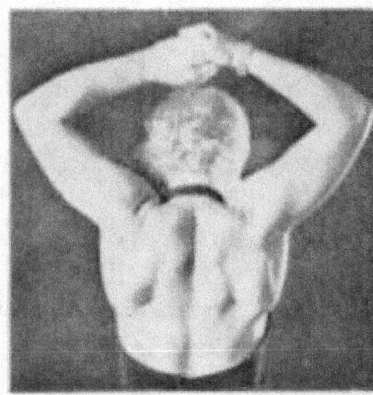

This young lady is a professional strong woman. When tensed, the muscles on her back stand out in bold relief, yet her physique is smooth and feminine when the muscles are in repose. Her professional name is Stout Lims.

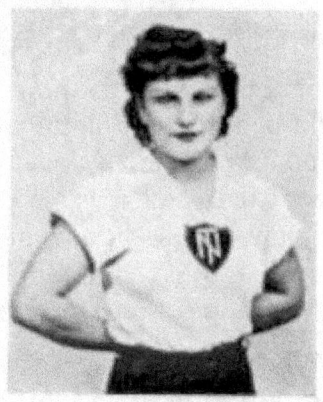

Jenny Catats, national gymnastic champion, one of our good friends of the 1936 Olympic trip. Although a very strong little girl, with style on the apparatus which compares favorably with the best masculine performers, she presents a very feminine and attractive appearance.

I ask them if they have harmony in their home lives; whether there is nagging, picking or fighting at meal times—for if these conditions are present it is better not to eat at all—and if they masticate their food thoroughly. It's especially important for the ambitious strength and health seeker to chew each bite of food as long as it can be retained in the mouth. Practically all strong men are deliberate eaters. It's difficult to tell whether they became strong because they eat slowly and carefully or whether being strong developed for them a tranquillity of mind, a placidness of disposition, a good nature, which results in turn in perfect digestion.

I ask them if they sleep soundly and well; how much and under what sort of conditions. We learned in the army that it pays to spend another ten minutes making a good bed as this would result in hours of additional, sound, restful sleep. Sleep is one of the important rules of health. If all of these rules are followed and the additional instructions this book contains are carefully observed, there is no reason why any man who is ambitious, willing to work for more strength and muscle, should not obtain it. There are some who have ideas of their own, who believe that they know best, who try to follow the advice of too many, rather than that of one qualified instructor, who will obtain only a partial measure of the results they should get.

Men with big bones will obtain large measurements faster than the light-boned man. But the man with light bones will have the more attractive physique, the more shapely limbs. That is one of the chief reasons for the undying fame of Eugene Sandow. He had comparatively small bones and when his arms were covered with a great deal of shapely muscle, his appearance was wonderful to behold.

There have been a few men who became quite strong without a great deal in the way of arm development. But I believe, without exception, these are men who never at any time specialized in arm development. There are others, who spend nearly all their training time at curling or chinning in an endeavor to build big arms, who receive only mediocre results for their pains. It requires a combination of heavy and moderate work, of intense and easier training, of arm specialization and rest periods to build the best arms. Of the very strong men I know who have arms small in proportion to their great strength, Bob Dudley, the tall young sailor who won the bent press championship in the middleweight class this year, one of the first men to bent press my big stage bell and to perform a one arm jerk with it too, when it was loaded to 217 pounds, is one. He's a good hand balancer and an all around lifter. Yet his arm was less than fifteen inches. Roy Hall of the Toronto-York weight lifting team has two hand snatched 250 pounds at a body weight of less than 180 pounds. He one hand clean and jerked 215 pounds. Yet he did not have a fifteen inch arm. Imperfections in his teeth held back his progress and he gained rapidly in weight and muscular size after having several infected teeth removed. Joe Mills, the Central Falls, Rhode Island, contender for the 132 pound title, has pressed 205 pounds in military style and his arm is just 13 inches. There was a British lifter, W. L. Carquest, one of the most famous lightweight lifters, who bent pressed 196 pounds when his upper arm measured only 13M2 inches. He specialized in this lift and although it is a good Triceps developer, there are, as our discussion of anatomy proved, many other muscles and muscle groups in the upper arm which must be developed to build bulk. J. H. Holliday of Manchester, England, went him one better, having only a inch arm and bent pressing 203.

Gord Venables, one of the best light-heavyweight and heavyweight lifters in North America, a place winner year after year in national competition, member of the world's championship team of 1937, champion of North America in his bodyweight class on several occasions, has a fifteen inch arm, which is not equal to the rest of his really magnificent physique. But I have never seen Gord practice even for a moment any sort of exercises, especially not those which" would result in greater arm development. He is a lifting specialist, has a fine body, but could stand a bit more in arm development. The most recent new senior national A. A. U. champion who has just been crowned, Elwood Kaufmann, in the 126 pound class, has very little arm development, and once again we have a case of a man who does not practice arm developing exercises.

The records of our pupils and the subjects of many of our self-improvement stories contain stories of lifters who have spent some time at dumbell work and greatly improved their development and muscular size, particularly the size of their arms. Emerson Bouyea of Bristol, Conn., a young man who was trying to recover from an operation for hernia when he first wrote to me and soon after took up York Bar Bell and Dumbell training, body weight 127 pounds, recently established three New England records in his class in lifting—190 press, 216 snatch and 281 clean and jerk. He practiced an all around program of bar bells and dumbells, not only overcame his original physical deficiency, greatly increased his strength and lifting power but immensely increased the size of his arm and other measurements as well. His is a case of a man who was so anxious to star at weightlifting that for a considerable period he concentrated only on weight-lifting movements and failed to gain in lifting ability, strength and development. Then he went back to including dumbell training in his program, and up his records soared rapidly. Jack Russel of London, Ont., some years ago the best lightweight lifter in the far-flung British Empire, a lifting specialist, spent some time with dumbell training, quickly increased his body weight to 165 pounds, his strength and lifting ability in proportion. There are numerous examples of the body builders, the exercise men, who included lifting motion exercises with their bar bell and dumbell training and registered immediate and pleasing gains—just further proof that the men who gain most, who have the greatest strength and the finest developed bodies, especially the arms, are those who practice an all around program, lifting, exercising with bar bells, dumbells and other apparatus, perhaps hand balancing too. Thus they build the muscles from every possible angle, develop as many of the 4,000,000,000 muscular fibres as they can and develop magnificent arms.

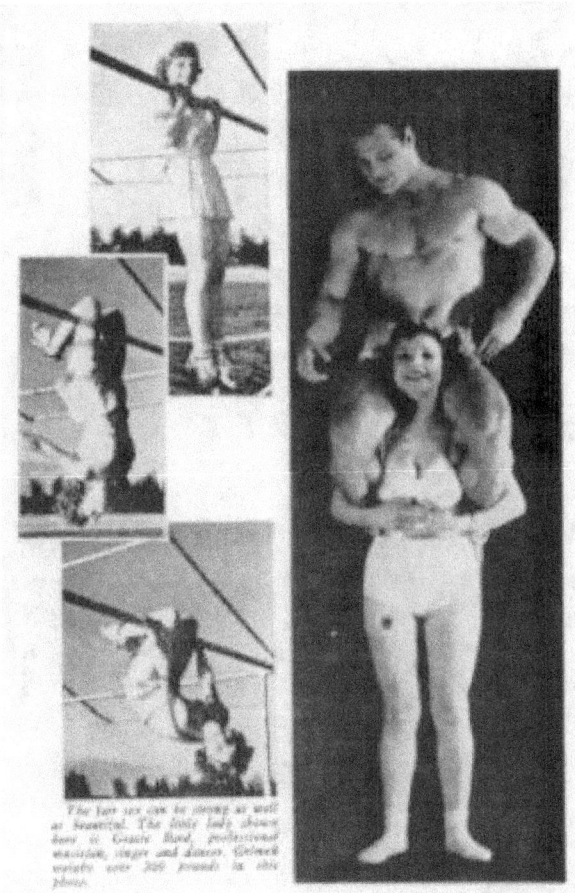

The fair sex can be strong as well as beautiful. The little lady shown here is Gracie Bard, professional acrobat, singer and dancer. Gracie weighs over 200 pounds in this photo.

Each man must be his own trainer to a certain degree. He must make a study of the methods usually practiced in obtaining the best arms, and if his own arm fails to respond to the training as outlined, if it is obstinate and he seems to make little progress toward his cherished goal of really impressive appearing arms, he must endeavor to determine just what he is doing that is wrong in his particular case. An intelligent study, a fair analysis of his training for greater arm size and strength and then some changes in his training program, following advice this book offers, should be the means of realizing his ambition.

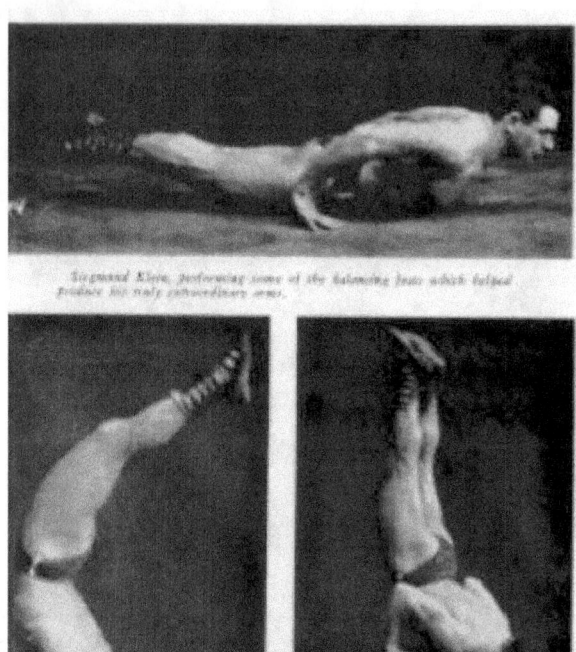

Siegmund Klein, performing some of the balancing feats which helped produce his truly extraordinary arms.

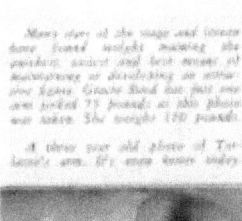

Many days of the sunny and lonely hours found weight making the youthful ardent and best means of incorporating or developing in other ways begin Grace had his just one arm jerked 75 pounds at this phase and when Sht weighs 180 pounds.

A three year old photo of Tallaret's arm. It's even better today.

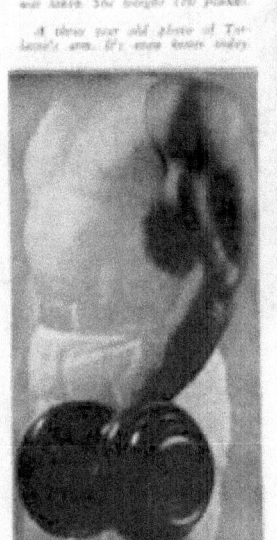

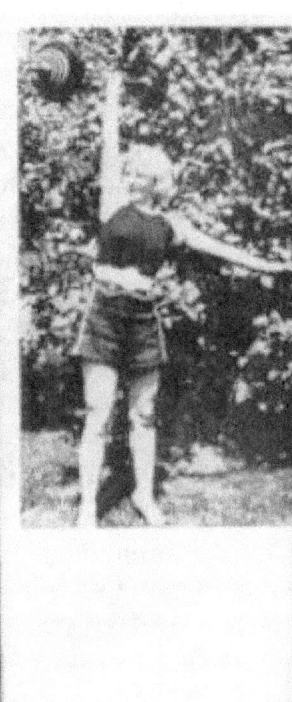

An arm that is thin and stringy is too often the result of too much ambition. It may be the effect of increasing the poundages in each exercise too rapidly. This not only cuts down the number of repetitions but causes considerable " cheating " with each movement, causing the body to do considerable of the work which should have been performed by the arms to obtain the best results. Increasing the poundages more rapidly than development can keep pace with it will usually result in a hard, thin and stringy arm. The arm, next to the neck, I believe, is the easiest part of the body to develop. It will improve rapidly, but of course it can not do the impossible.

Variation, usually termed irregular training, is offered with the York Bar Bell courses to prevent a condition such as I describe. There is the limit day during which the student endeavors to work up to or beyond his best of the past. On that day some form of repetitions of each particular exercise for the arms should be practiced—the famous "York Heavy and Light System" which I believe is original in my courses. As usually performed a weight is selected in each movement which permits seven or eight movements. Immediately the weight is reduced by the degree which practice has proven to be necessary in your particular case—usually about twenty per cent. Immediately seven or eight additional movements of the same exercise are practiced. One of the best ways to train with dumbells and the " Heavy and Light System " is to have two sets of dumbells, one loaded for the first or heavier poundage, the other for the light. On this limit day, the tendons, ligaments and muscles are strengthened. Not so much is obtained in bulk as in strength. However, the heavy day in connection with more moderate days of training will invariably bring the desired effect.

As few as five or six movements of a particular exercise will bring very little in the way of favorable results. A fair number of movements are necessary to break down muscular tissue and to bring the blood rushing to the rescue of the working part with its load of new replacement and building material. To obtain best results this blood must be kept in the part being exercised for a considerable period so that it has time to do its work well. We prefer to avoid very high repetitions—not passing fifteen except in movements such as the shoulder shrug, the raise on toes or others which are quite easy; for a weight is too light which can be handled more than fifteen repetitions. It will result in the tough, stringy muscles I am writing about—muscles not unlike those obtained by the marathon runner, or the tennis player who regularly follows the large tournaments and is frequently extended to five hard sets. On one of the usual three training days a week I advocate the selection of a weight which will permit fifteen movements. This develops endurance to a considerable degree, as well as muscular size and shape. On the third day of training I suggest the selection of a weight which allows ten movements. This develops strength to a great degree, and bulk. Our muscles have the habit of being in ruts, accustomed to the work they are asked to do. It is nature's way to build the muscles so that they can perform the work required of them and a bit more. But this irregular training must be practiced to cause these muscles to change their habits, to get out of the rut in which they have been operating.

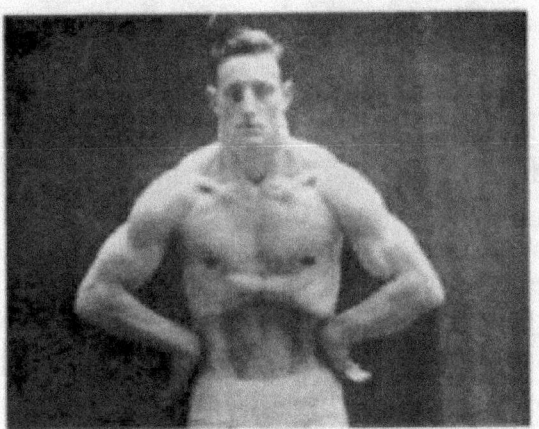

The system of irregular training I briefly described has brought sensational results. All around training, avoiding the use of the muscles in the same groove always, but building and strengthening them from every possible angle through the practice of a wide variety of exercises will bring you best results as it has brought success to others in the past.

Last year, before my annual birthday event, I followed a similar sort of training—Saturday, always our limit day, lift all I could. With bent pressing it is not wise to have two other rather severe training days so I bent pressed on

Wednesday, as a rule, not quite my limit. Exercised on Monday, going through the course of exercises offered in my book, " How To Be Strong, Healthy and Happy," two separate times. These exercises are not unlike the exercises in the York Bar Bell courses, except that there are twelve of them instead of ten. As in the York courses, the first course includes the front curl, the second the back curl, the first the regular press, the second the press behind neck, the first the deep knee bend on toes, the second the deep knee bend flat-footed, the first the regular dead lift, the second the stiff-legged dead lift, etc., somewhat similar exercises but performed in a slightly different manner—exercises which brought fine results as proven by my lifting of November, 1938, which is now history.

In recent years my training time had been little, usually Saturday being my one opportunity. But a few weeks before my annual birthday contest I managed to train at least four times a week. I have a fondness for the bent press and at my annual lifting show of 1936 I had bent pressed the Cyr dumbell weighing 202 pounds. The next year, 1937, I had pressed my big stage bell officially for the first time and it weighed 220 pounds. But last year I made a modern world's record in the bent press with a lift of 263% pounds, weighed on a tested platform scale with competent officials serving as weighers—notably Jack Ayres of Wilmington, Delaware, athletic commissioner of the state of Delaware, and long a member of the Middle Atlantic A. A. U. weight lifting committee. He is a weight lifting enthusiast of long standing and was one of the officials who served when I won the amateur heavyweight title in 1927. Another one was Joe Ortolini of Rochester, New York, the weight lifting coach of the Y. M. C. A. of that city, a man who has seldom missed a weight lifting contest in these United States east of Chicago in many years. The other official weigher was Lou Schell of York. A considerable group of spectators, who were invited to look at the poundage, came forward and saw the scale balanced at $263^1/2$.

This improvement proves two things: First that I practice what I preach, have obtained good results from the training methods I offer to you who read this book, and to my pupils throughout the world, men of 44 countries, who number more than 100,000 at present; and second that I " know whereof I speak." The methods I advocate will bring results. They have produced more outstanding physical specimens than every system of training offered to the strength and health seeking public before or since. They revolutionized physical training. Over ten thousand testimonials have been received, and it's one of my greatest pleasures to contemplate the physical improvement so many men have made—the overcoming of illness, injuries, paralysis, heart and lung troubles, rupture, bad stomachs, and of course the simpler ills of constipation, indigestion, etc. It's been a pleasure to be in this work of showing others how to be strong, healthy and happy. I am glad that I have the rest of my life to spend at this game of weight lifting which has meant so much to me and will be the means of helping so many others—of building the youth of our nation so that America will always be a stronghold of brave and strong men.

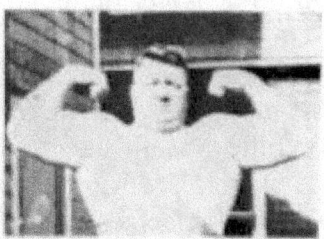

In my enthusiasm I branched off a bit from the subject at the beginning of this chapter. I sought to prove that all around training brings best results. I built my arm to 17% inches at the completion of my now famous, special twenty weeks' training. In the beginning it had never exceeded 16 inches. Later it stretched the tape to a full \ fVz inches. Although I did not specialize in arm developing exercises during that period, I did build the ability to perform a correct back hand curl of 140 pounds, which at that time was a record and to my knowledge has only been exceeded by big Dave Mayor's 145. And Dave is a physical giant,— is the possessor of the largest muscular arms in the world and is the best man at the rowing motion I have ever seen.

For the first three months of this training I followed the York courses exactly as they are offered to every pupil: On alternate training days, rest day in between each—Course No. i consisting of a warming up exercise, ten bar bell and seven dumbell exercises. The next training day—York Course No. 3, weight lifting exercises. And this course is the one which brought the best results. Rapid press, rapid bouncing deep knee bend, repetition one hand snatch, one hand jerk, repetition or dead hang snatches, dead hang cleans and repetition jerks, rapid dead lifts and, perhaps best of all, rapid rowing motions. For this exercise which permits the handling of very heavy weights—170 ten repetitions in my case, 200 ten repetitions for big Dave—develops more muscular bulk and strength than any exercise I know. It particularly builds the deep lying muscle you learned of in the chapter on anatomy, the Brachialis Amicus, a muscle lying under the Biceps, really between the Biceps and the Triceps. When the Brachialis Anticus swells or grows, the bulk of the arm increases rapidly. This muscle will receive little benefit and less development from the usual Biceps exercises, curling and chinning. It will receive little benefit from Triceps exercises, pressing and dipping. But it does obtain considerable benefit with resulting development from the rowing motion, the cleans, snatches, rapid dead lifts, pulling the weight high at the finish, the one hand snatch—all reasons why York Course No. 3, without specialization in arm development, will build wonderful arms. Examine the arms of the York lifters which appear with two of the charts in this book. They depict magnificent development and not one of these men has specialized in arm development. Those great arms are solely the product of training for lifting and competitive lifting. Course No. 2 next and then Course No. 4, the weight lifting course. Every eight days I completed the four courses and would start again with Course No. 1.

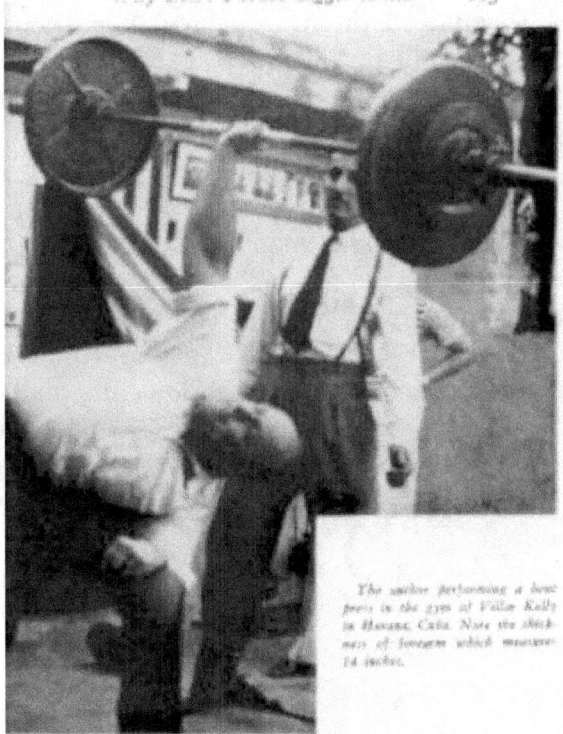

The author performing a bent press in the gym of Villar Kelly in Havana, Cuba. Note the thickness of forearm which measures 14 inches.

It has frequently been a source of disappointment to the average body builder when he looks in the mirror at his undersized arms, after a great deal of hard work, specializing in exercises which were designed to build the arms, and then to see the beautiful, the magnificent, the shapely, powerful and swelling Biceps of the lifting specialist—the man who has practiced repetition exercises to develop his lifting ability. For, as mentioned before, the man who lifts only with single attempts on the lifts will become strong but will not have the resulting development to match his ability.

The ideal program for developing the arm and the entire body is an all around program with a heavy day weekly, two fairly heavy days and one or two light or tinkering days. During the last eight weeks of my special twenty weeks' training I specialized on lifting three days weekly, and performed rather heavy dumbell exercise on the two remaining training days a week. There was considerable of the rowing motion, both upright and leaning, single and double one hand curls, alternate curl and press, the twisting curl or Zottman exercise, the curls performed both upright and leaning with one hand upon a box, and a host of other movements. This diversified all around program brought me results—a forearm of more than 14 inches and a Biceps which extended to 17V2 as before mentioned and unusual ability on the quick as well as the slow lifts and strength feats. It reorganized my entire physical nomenclature and made me the really big fellow I am today with a bodyweight which hovers around the 250 pound mark while in good condition.

If You Fail to Get Results

THERE was considerable in the last chapter for the benefit of those ambitious arm builders who have failed to obtain the size and bulk they so greatly desire to build. There is much to the subject so we will continue.

Make haste slowly. If you find that your rate of growth in strength and development does not keep pace with the double progressive system as you are following it, do not increase the weight and the repetitions for a time. Rather than to go on trying to force too rapid growth and retarding your progress in the process, take your time. Be patient. Some men gain very rapidly. For the first few weeks in my special training, my clean and jerk record increased five pounds weekly, until the stage was reached where it hovered near the same point for a number of weeks. Each man, as I wrote before, must be his own trainer to a great degree, for only he knows how he feels, only he can determine whether he is training too hard or not enough.

I find it wise to work on nerve just once a week—for demands must be made so that nature will answer those increased demands with more endurance, greater strength and larger development. The other nights of the week it is best to carefully avoid training on one's nerve. Do not perform the last five or six movements with clenched teeth, straining, working on your nerve to reach the allotted number of counts; and don't confuse laziness with working on your nerve. You'll have to be the best judge of that—to know whether it is working on your nerve or just an antipathy toward extending yourself on that particular day. Remember, please, you will obtain better results by training, not straining. You must exert yourself to the limit at times, then train more moderately, performing the exercises correctly on other training days.

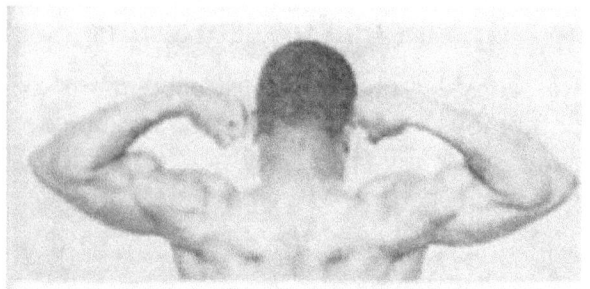

Arm development of John Terry, United States 132 pound champion and world record holder. Terry has extremely long arms, so well developed that they appear very muscular as shown here. He holds the world's record on the dead weight lift at 383 pounds.

Tom Tyler, a famous cine hero movie star. He was U. S. heavyweight lifting champion when this photo was made.

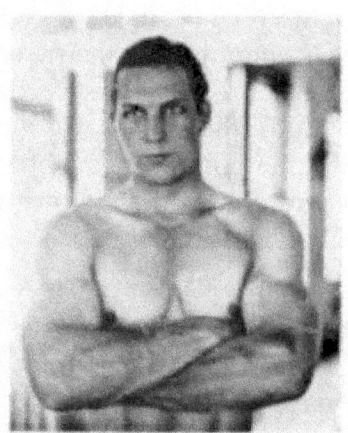

You gentlemen who are readers of Strength and Health Magazine, especially the department devoted to the American Strength and Health League, must have been impressed with the fact that more men win gold medals for performing eighteen consecutive chins than in any other way. The devotees of the chinning exercise are legion. So many men believe that this is all that is necessary to develop a good arm. But how often do you see one of these chinners who has a good arm? Like my own arm, early in my training career, when I had the burning ambition to be strong and an athletic champion, when I was six feet, three inches tall and weighed all of 150 pounds soaking wet, when I would display the little hump on my upper arm, my older and stronger brothers always laughingly called it my " manufactured bump." I had to manufacture them some way, for I didn't have them naturally, having weighed just 140 pounds when I first reached my present height of six feet three. I was thin enough that I came pretty close to the necessity of standing twice in one place to cast a shadow.

But joking aside, the chinners rarely have good arms, and what you have read in preceding chapters must be giving you a more than good inkling ol just why they do not. The. upper arm is designed primarily to perform two motions, curl and press. Many young men believe that the floor press and the two hands chin are sufficient to build their arms, but the lack of results they receive is the best proof that there are other ways of building good arms. Years ago one to five pound dumbells were advocated by the leading trainers of the day. Sandow was responsible for this in the beginning, I believe. While he had developed his own physique first by lifting and wrestling, later by professional stage work with the hardest kind of lifting, later in life he issued a physical culture course, the apparatus of which consisted of three and five pound spring dumbells. He sought to prove to the public that his strength and matchless physique were the result of training with this very light equipment, when all students of physical training know well that he performed the hardest kind of lifting and supporting feats. In one part of his act he made a bent press with a huge bar bell consisting of two large spheres. At the completion of the lift, the dumbell would be opened and there were two attractive young ladies who had provided the weight to be lifted. His record in the bent press was 271 pounds. In his act he carried a small horse at extended straight arms across the stage. He performed many outstanding lifting and supporting feats in the many years during which he was a professional performer. This of course was responsible for his outstanding development. Nevertheless, when I made my beginning in physical training, five pound dumbells, wooden Indian clubs, and wands were the means of developing muscles offered to the physical culturist of that day thirty years ago. The exercises were posed for by strength athletes, such as Sandow, men who had obtained their development through the hardest kind of training. Many years of my life went by with endeavors to obtain better development with these light methods. I built a certain form of endurance but only the manufactured bumps my older brothers laughed at.

During the period I have been discussing the athletes of the day went in for repetition lifting of many sorts. I remember their photos so well. Many of them had about the same development one finds today with the marathon runners who cover their twenty-six miles and some odd yards. Usually they are about as big as a minute and look as if a fair breeze would blow them away; for constant repetitions with light weights reduce the size of the limbs, make them thin, stringy and tough and particularly hard to develop. Well do I remember the bony appearance of the world's champion at bag punching a few years ago. Attired as he was in the popular turtle neck sweater of the day, I could see that he had an arm which appeared little larger than my wrist and through his heavy trousers I could see the hip bones protruding like the bones of some poor old worn-out horse. And his shoulders reminded one best of the hooks in a clothes closet. I devoured every book on physical training I could obtain—and there were many in those days. I lived near the Carnegie Library and spent a good share of my time over there. I have a retentive memory and I well remember the photos I saw thirty years ago, especially of the strength and athletic stars of the day. The accounts of the early Olympic games are indelibly stamped in my memory as if they occurred but yesterday. I read these books so thoroughly that I will never forget the types of physiques which were shown there. I remember the heavy physiques of men like Cyclops, Launcester Elliot and Fred

Winters—one of the first Olympic lifters,—of Steinbach and Demetros Tofalas, who also competed in the Olympic games. I can mentally visualize the anger Steinbach displayed when they would not let him lift at the Athens Olympics of 1896, ruling that he was a professional; and his contempt as he later went over and easily continentalled and jerked the weight others had struggled with, then disdainfully hurled it to the ground and walked away.

And I can see just as plainly the sort of physiques the men who held the endurance lifting records during the last part of the 19th century and the beginning of the twentieth possessed. Max Dantage of Vienna performed the deep knee bend 6,000 times in four hours June 4th, 1899. His leg development reminded me a lot of the arm possessed by the better developed men. The men I first mentioned were huge and powerful; they had obtained results from their heavy lifting, but did not practice a variety of movements to improve their physiques and were far too corpulent. The men who practiced repetitions had thin stringy muscles like the before mentioned marathoner. Ed G. Stickney at Lynn, Mass., elevated a 4 pound dumbell 6,000 times in just a few seconds less than one hour, back in 1885. And all he got for his pains was just the ability to lift 4 pounds 6,000 times— nothing in the way of development. It's nature's way to build the strength or endurance to perform the tasks asked of the muscles. Progressive training makes it possible to do the work asked. But if progression as in the case of the marathoner consists only of running a bit more each day, until the full twenty-six miles can be covered, only endurance is created. And if a man's ambition is to see how many times he can deep knee bend with no resistance or elevate a five or ten pound dumbell, he'll just develop the ability to make more repetitions. It does not require strength or muscle to lift five or ten pounds—a child can do it—and muscles of a child's size will result from these high repetitions. The heavy single attempts of the huge continental lifters produced big bodies, powerful limbs, strong tendons, but not an attractive physique. A combination of exercises, heavy and more moderate, and some specialization to properly shape and mould all the parts of the body are required.

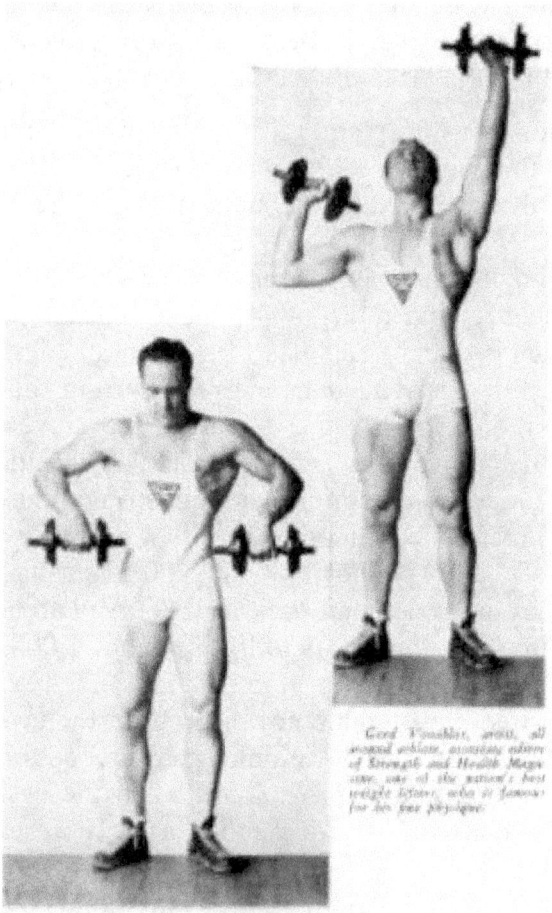

Gord Venabler, artist, all around athlete, associate editor of Strength and Health Magazine, was one of the nation's best weight lifters, who is famous for his fine physique.

H. Pennock holds the record in pressing a ten pound dumbell. He set the mark at 8,431 repetitions in 1870. It took him four hours and thirty-four minutes to make the record. Another American, A. Corcoran of Chicago, made an even better record by " putting up" a 12 pound dumbell an even 14,000 times in 1873.

Other repetition lifting such as the 36 times that Louis Cyr lifted 162V2 pounds from floor to overhead with one arm would produce considerable strength—as would the lifting of a 100 pound dumbell 27 times from the shoulder by William Conture who only weighed 149 pounds. Henry Saltiel elevated a 71V2 pound dumbell 118 times, changing hands with each lift. Anthony McKinley of Philadelphia was another who went in for repetition lifting with light dumbells, succeeding with hoisting a dumbell weighing 10 pounds 1V2 ounces 10,000 times. When C. O. Breed lifted a barrel from the floor weighing 201V2 pounds 240 times in ten minutes, he performed a feat which required unusual gripping power as well as endurance. G. W. Roche of San Francisco lifted a 25 pound dumbell 450 times from the shoulder.

While most of the old timers went in for repetition lifting with light weights, there were a few really strong men who entered contests in repetition lifting,—succeeding with high repetitions on some very heavy weights. These men would receive good results for their efforts, but the men who lifted very light weights thousands of times only developed a certain form of endurance, endurance which would probably serve them in no way other than repetition pressing with a light weight.

To practice any form of high repetition exercises, chinning, curling, dipping or pressing will bring the Biceps to a certain degree of toughness and endurance, but there is no proof that it will bring even a fair degree of muscular size and development.

Others fail to build their arms to the desired point because they perform too many arm exercises. They may use satisfactory poundages, the proper number of repetitions, and perform the exercises correctly enough and still not obtain good results from practicing too many arm exercises in each training period. Some men can stand more than others. After a considerable period of striving for super arm development, you can easily measure your gains or lack of gains with the tape and with the weight handled. If you can continue to progress with a system of a great many arm exercises, by all means continue that method. But if you are not making reasonable progress, try something else. Moderate your training efforts, not performing more than five arm exercises in a single exercise period; or try the system of exercising the arms considerably every training day one week, and the following week no arm exercises except the regular exercises in one of the courses. The third week go back again to arm specialization and then moderate rest for the arms the fourth week, etc.

There are men who have received favorable results from exercising the upper body only one week and the lower body only another week. The object of course is to keep the bulk of the blood in the upper part of the body one week and the lower the next—to make great demands on just one part of the body, to be sure that that part is well nourished and supplied with rebuilding material by the blood. After a considerable period of double progressive training for the arms, you can provide variation by adopting one of the various different styles of training I will suggest in this volume.

Too many arm exercises at a single training period may make such demands upon the arm muscles that the re-plenishing function of the blood is temporarily over-whelmed, having all it can do to replace the material used rather than to provide a surplus for growth. A failure to grow in size is good proof that the arm is being overworked.

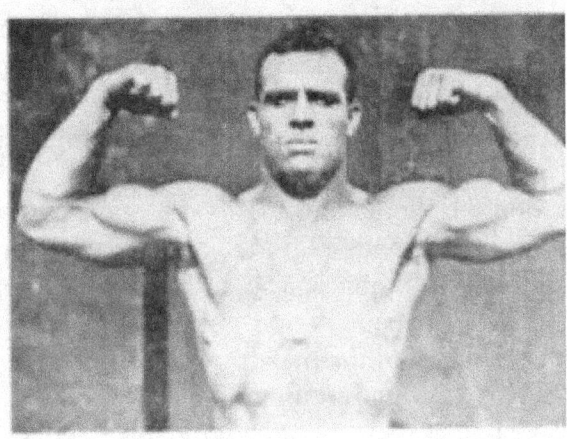

There is a great deal of difference in humans concerning the amount of work they can perform and the amount of fatigue they can withstand. Some men recuperate quickly while others take days or weeks to recover from overwork. Perfect functioning organs make possible rapid recuperation.

There are many men who experience a long period of enforced labor and become so fatigued that it will take them days to recover. An animal can be chased by dogs until it drops dead from exhaustion, and there have been so many cases of driving a horse during a period of emergency so that it dropped dead at the finish. It was not heart failure which caused their demise, but fatigue poisoning. Fatigue in the arm while practicing a great number of arm movements is a mild form of this fatigue poisoning. Fatigue poisoning is often called " replacement of waste " by prominent physiologists. Some men have the ability to replace this waste more rapidly and more completely than others. Experience will teach you how you feel after a long training period. If you have a feeling of exhilaration an hour later, or in any event are not unduly tired the next day, you are not exercising too much.

Fatigue poisons take place for two reasons: One, the inability of the blood to carry off the waste products of exertion and to replace them with fresh building and operating materials. And the other is what is known as an oxygen debt. Oxygen is required to form combustion with the food properties carried by the blood stream, and during great exertion the blood can not absorb and carry as much of the oxygen as the body requires. This first causes breath-lessness, later great fatigue through the prolonged exertion. A period of rest or recuperation is required to pay off this oxygen debt and permit all parts of the body to operate normally again. Through training, the processes of the body are improved to an extent that wind and endurance are better.

Absolute collapse, after driving oneself for a long period in a race, will never occur through weight training. Fatigue poisoning may be felt to a much lesser degree. You are the best judge of whether you have a feeling of lassitude through overtraining, or through wrong living of some sort. If it is the former, moderate your efforts until such a time as an improvement in the latter has given you better operating functions, better respiration, better circulation, better digestion, assimilation and elimination.

The limit in the case of one man may be a great deal more or less than that of another. The men who have obtained best results in physical training are more often those men who are healthy, possess good recuperative powers, and can train for hours each day without a feeling of fatigue the next day. I know many champions who would train three or four hours a day during the period when they were most enthusiastic. Dave Mayor would train an hour in the morning, an hour in the afternoon, and another hour or two in the evening. He was most interested in lifting and would spend an hour at pressing, an hour at snatching and his evening session at performing the two hands clean and jerk.

There are other men like Steve Stanko, present heavyweight champion, who train very little and still obtain sensational results. Both of these young men, while quite slender—120 pounds at a height of approximately six feet with both of them—had powerful masculine forebears before them. Heredity played its part to a great measure in their cases. Big Dave Mayor more than doubled his weight after he reached his present height. Stanko increased his weight by a hundred pounds. Steve Stanko makes a few lifts on Monday and Wednesday, spends a bit more time on Saturday, and became one of the world's best heavyweights in less than a year since he was first heard of. If you have such perfect operation of organs, such potential power, you are fortunate. If you do not have, you must work harder and longer.

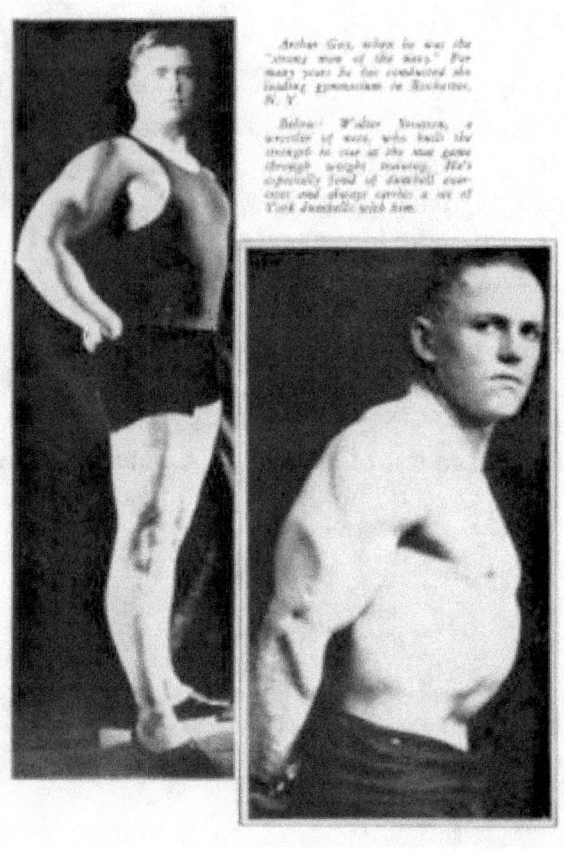

I have not been able to cover all possible cases. But to summarize what I have written—if you get good results with the methods you are following continue with that system of training. You'll reach your goal in the end. But if your progress is unusually slow, or you don't get ahead at all, change your training methods. When a young man who works hard all day on the farm, a section or road gang, in the mines, asks me how he should train, I invariably suggest a system of practicing certain key exercises in groups of five. For instance: Select a weight which can be curled five times. Rest a while. Perform five more curls, rest again, and then another five. Go through the entire course in this manner. It does not require so much endurance; there are enough movements to draw the blood to the working muscle. Energy is conserved, yet the muscles will gain in size and shape as well as strength.

Fewer repetitions with heavy weights strengthen tendons and ligaments, toughen muscles, make it possible to succeed with more in a single lift. This is all necessary in physical training and this sort of training should be incorporated in the training system as we have suggested for Saturday. But there should be the other days in which ten to fifteen movements are practiced, to build muscular size and shape and a fair amount of endurance. Train, don't strain; be sure that you don't overtrain. Work hard, long and enthusiastically and you are sure to attain your goal of a great deal more than average arm strength and development.

Are Free Hand Exercises of Value?

We have considered the arm anatomically, we have discussed the world's largest armed men, covered considerable of training methods, reasons for failure to obtain the big arms desired, and now we arc ready to reflect upon exercise of the arms—the means of obtaining the arm size, strength and shapeliness every body builder desires.

I know you want bigger arms. That's the paramount reason why you are reading this book. Just what means should you select to obtain them? Should you practice free hand exercises, or, among the other non-apparatus exercises, chinning, dipping, resisting one muscle against the other? Will you obtain sufficient arm size and strength through the practice of some athletic sport? And if experience has shown you that you can not hope to obtain the strength and development you desire without employing some form of apparatus as a developing medium just what equipment will you select?

There are a number of well-known appliances to consider: The Giant Crusher Grip, designed to develop the crushing muscles of the body—muscles which are difficult

to reach in any other manner. The Iron Shoe, designed to build strength in ligaments, tendons and arms. While its movement is restricted it does build the bending and break-ing power of the body. Cables, more commonly called Chest Expanders—universally used and have proven to develop extraordinary Triceps in particular. Dumbells, which permit a greater variety of movement and more satisfactory progression than any of the methods we have mentioned. But not light dumbells. Weights heavy enough to exert the muscle groups involved in each particular exer-cise so that they can be exercised in accord with the prin-ciples already mentioned in this book. Heavy and light system of the limit day of training, ten repetitions one training day and the use of a poundage which allows fifteen movements another day of the week.

And bar bells which permit the practice of weight lifting and weight lifting exercises make possible the handling of very heavy weights, without which the ultimate in strength and development can not be obtained. They make possible the building of really good arms in less time, and with less effort. As our discussion progresses, I believe you will agree that the best results are had when " all three " (bar bells, dumbells and cables) are incorporated in the weekly training periods. Variety adds interest to the exercising program. It causes you to look forward with pleasurable enthusiasm to the next period of training. It brings into play a great many more muscles, gets you out of the tut of just curling and pressing and strengthens the muscles as well as developing them from every possible angle.

Hundreds of fine exercises are possible when the strength seeker has the equipment above enumerated to use when he desires.

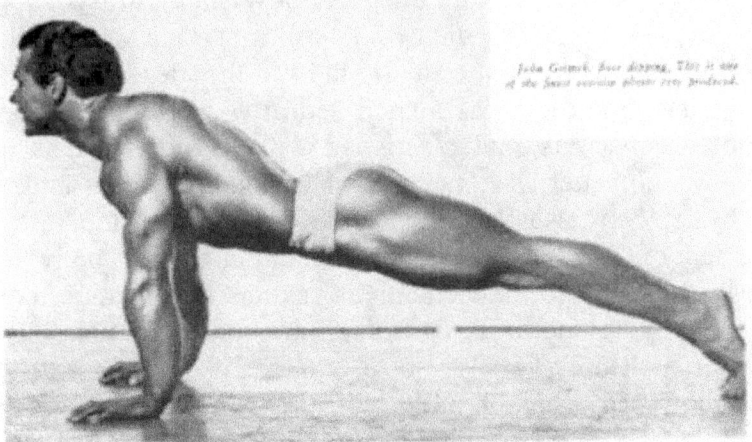

First we will consider the non-apparatus methods. I have always written that any exercise is better than no exercise. I should qualify that statement a bit by saying that any

117

vigorous exercise, which follows principles of training which have proven to be good, is better than no exercise. For arm waving, as is considered exercise by the uninitiated, requires more in the way of an expenditure of energy than it produces. When we were children in school the physical director would come to each classroom in turn and have us go through these arm waving exercises. It did break the monotony; it did provide interest and relaxation; with many it inculcated a desire to go farther into physical training. But as far as muscle building was concerned the efforts expended were nil. Muscles are made only when they are asked or forced to overcome resistance. The greater the effort demanded of them, providing the rules of health are followed, will result in larger muscular development. I qualify this statement, for we know of many men who, when they work at all, must earn their few dollars as day laborers, usually pick and shovel men, who are thin, scrawny and have no noticeable development. Some of them have a toughness of the muscles which permits them to keep going all day, but the thin scrawny muscles they own would not be desired by any physical culturist. There are powerful, healthy men who perform hard labor. And the difference between the two is the life they lead. One man obtains good food, has a good bed in which to sleep, does not dissipate, is rather satisfied with his lot because he knows no better. The man who is little more than a shadow physically is usually a man who dissipates to the fullest extent of his pocketbook and the endurance of his body. He robs his body of the elements it requires by spending most of his money on drink or worse forms of dissipation. Hard effort will only be a strain to him, for nature has little or nothing with which to build.

Any unbiased authority will admit that progressive apparatus is the best training medium, because exactly the weight or other form of resistance (as in devices using a number of springs or cables) can be employed to provide the proper resistance for the muscle group involved. Actual free hand movements will provide little benefit, because they are not intense enough,to develop muscle or to engender internal changes. Unless the man or woman who practices such methods is sadly out of condition, they can not even cause themselves to breathe faster through free hand movements, or even to perspire unless it is a hot day. Without an amplification of the breathing, a speeding up of respiration, enough exertion to improve appetite, digestion and elimination, exercise is almost completely valueless.

There have been, especially since the advent of the great Eugene Sandow, millions of men who desired to have muscles, strength and physical proportions like he had built for himself. At the close of the last century and the beginning of this, many train you by mail professors sprang up. I believe I am right in saying that, without exception, every one of these men obtained his greatest results in building the magnificent bodies they showed, by weight training. They may have used cables, wrestled, tumbled, handbalanced, but the lifting of weights brought their bodies above the average. And in the beginning of my interest in physical training, about 1909, we find these men offering various systems of non-apparatus courses. When I finally managed to delve to the bottom of the training methods of the greatest physical specimens, which was in 1923, there were many training methods being offered to the strength and development seeking public.

There was Earle Liederman, who at that time led them all in volume of business and enrollments, who offered cables to his advanced pupils. Siegmund Breitbart had a spring, not unlike our Crusher Grip of today, as the sole equipment he offered. Antone Matysek, who like the others had developed one of the most magnificent bodies in the world, offered a leverage affair, which, while having more opportunity for exertion than some of the others, was restricted in movement. There was Titus, who offered non-apparatus exercises. Swoboda had ceased to advertise, but had claimed that his great strength and muscle had been developed through the means of muscle tensing. Sandow was still alive, offering his spring dumbells. Charles Atlas was just beginning, offering non-apparatus exercises and " knocking " weights with all his might and main so that he could sell his own course. As he once told me, " If I don't knock weights I can't sell my course, and I find it hard enough to sell as it is." Strongfort was a big advertiser then—exercises without apparatus to some pupils and weights to those who took his advanced course. There was Farmer Burns—wrestling, of course. Benny Leonard who, having been a boxer, naturally intended to use boxing methods. Otto Arco, who certainly was one of the most muscular men who ever lived and a very good personal friend of mine, had developed an apparatus light in weight, which developed the muscles through balance. Zbyszko who taught wrestling. And many, many others. Scores of others.

Tony Terlazzo, world's champion and world's record holder.

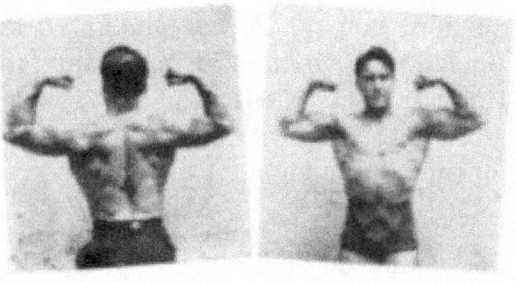

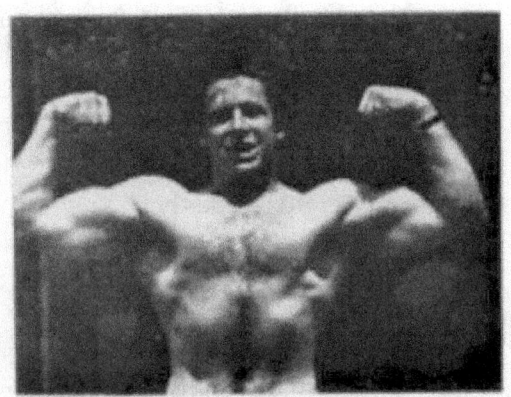

The United States Heavyweight lifting champion of 1937 and 1938. Believed to be the strongest man in America at present.

With the possible exception of Benny Leonard, former world's boxing champion, these men had all used weights in their training. Why then did they not offer the means of training which had brought such good results to them? I believe the sole reason was the fact that they found it was not possible to operate a mail order muscle business with the moderate profit the sale of weights permitted. With a bar bell set, there is a lot of expensive equipment to supply. With the York Big Ten Special, for instance, there are the knurled steel bar, heavy duty collars, special hold-titc collars, the dumbell bars, eight more collars and a wrench; a variety of plates ranging in weight from 1 Vl to 50 with the 310 pound set, 24 plates in all; the machining, painting, packing; the head strap and chain, the wrist developer, the Iron Boots, one of the finest mediums to develop the lower part of the body, the three leg courses, the four dumbell courses, the four bar bell and lifting courses, and personal instruction—not enough margin to operate a big office, spend thousands even hundreds of thousands annually for advertising, as did Earle Liederman, and still manage to keep ahead of the creditors.

So they had to think up reasons why the use of weights would not bring results or were actually harmful. When there was an endeavor at the Federal Trade Commission investigations to prove that Charles Atlas regularly trained with weights, his attorney would admit that he used them, yes. For hundreds of witnesses could be found who had seen him using them! And in the story of his own life he told of training with weights. But the lawyer would admit only that he used the weights to " demonstrate his strength." My reply to that was: " Our world's champions, Johnny Terpak and Tony Terlazzo, spend most of their time pounding typewriters. That is what really makes them strong enough to be world's weight lifting champions. Of course they do go out to the gymnasium three to five times a week and use weights, but only as a means of demonstrating the strength they developed through pounding the typewriter and to show the other fellows the advantages of typewriter pounding as a training medium."

Fortunately nearly all of the " fakirs " have disappeared from the " train you by mail" business. Although as Barnum said, " There is one born every minute." Now with a greater birth rate there are at least two born every minute.

But there weren't enough to go around so many of them had to give up business. The ambitious body culturists are becoming more enlightened. They have found in their own cases and that of others that the only way to obtain satisfactory results is to work against resistance—that progressive resistance, training with apparatus like dumbells and bar bells which permit the increase of the poundages by small jumps as low as a pound and a quarter at a time, a weight that can hardly be felt, but does in time bring greater strength inside and out, with more muscle, or cables which permit the adding of one strand after another as strength increases, bring superior results. In any Y. M. C. A. or gymnasium there are men far better built than the average men who frequent those places, and the beginner in asking them how they got that way will invariably be informed that progressive training brought them from usually a frail beginning to their state of outstanding development. One man who receives exceptional results tells another. He takes up progressive training and tells still more. So this game of muscle building through progressive training is like the rolling snowball—the bigger it gets the faster it collects snow. The bigger the group of men who have obtained their hearts' desire through weight training, the faster new men learn of weights and other forms of progressive training, and succeed in reaching their physical goals.

Now that you are at least partially informed concerning the advantages of and the reasons for weight training, we will go on with our discussion of no apparatus training methods. After the arm waving movements there are various other exercises which bring into play body leverage. Of course these will bring better results than just the forms of free hand movements. During the great war, the machine shops and factories of our country were too busy making guns, bullets and other deadly appliances to supply thr millions of men in training with any form of training apparatus. So it was ncccssary to build the strength, endurance and agility of the soldiers with body resistance movements or with actual work. There were few soldiers who did not have an opportunity to wear a few blisters on their hands with pick and shovel. There were few who did not have long hikes carrying a surprising amount of equipment. And there were few who were not required to perform a great deal of additional heavy tasks. But there was physical training for all. There were a great variety of gun drills and although a gun weighed only about nine pounds, with high repetitions with each exercise a certain amount of benefit was obtained. The calisthenics with a gun, outside of the regular bayonet drill, consisted of movements not unlike bar bell training. Evidently the officer who had arranged the exercises was familiar with weight training, believed in it and did the best he could without a means of making the exercise progressive.

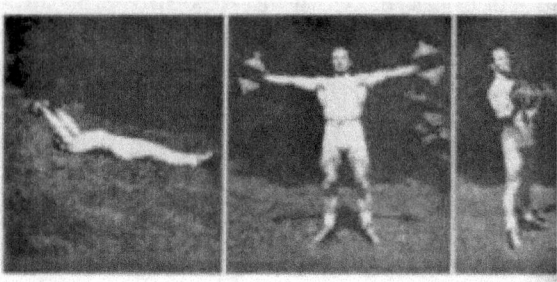

The Straddle Hop was one of the popular exercises. It's done with weights too and brings superior results. The soldier would stand in the position of attention, heels together, hands at sides. Then he would suddenly spread his feet, raising the hands and clapping them overhead simultaneously, then back to the starting position and continue this with a regular cadence for at least 32 counts. It was a good exercise; better with real resistance, but it did bring some results. Leg raising in various forms, sit ups, the inverted bicycle ride were other exercises designed to develop the mid-section. Ground dipping alone was practiced. And we had an acrobatically inclined officer who had us perform many other feats, the most notable of which was the dive and roll. We would dive and roll over first one man, then two, then three. The man who missed had to get down for the others to dive over and all would continue until the best managed to clear the backs of a dozen men.

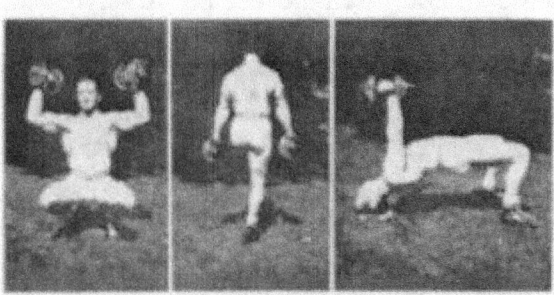

A miniature course of dumbbell exercises which develop all the major muscle groups of the body. Posed by Eddie Harrison.

One of the best exercises consisted of starting from the position of a soldier, bending over to touch the ground with palms of the hands without bending the knees if possible, then thrusting the legs back so that the back was straight, next dipping until the chest touched the sand, back to straight arms, legs back to their former position, then stand erect. About eight of such movements provided considerable in the way of exertion. There were many variations of this movement besides the really rugged games which were played. Break the camel's back was one of the most vigorous. Two sides were chosen. One side would get down on their hands and knees. The others would pile on one at a time, the idea being to leap on the backs with such force that the man underneath would flatten or fall to the side. Then the second group who were piling on to break the camel's back would win.

Such movements will serve when nothing better is available. It was the best means of training millions of men where apparatus is not available, but far superior results can be had by the body culturist training alone or with a friend or two and his modern apparatus.

The usual course without apparatus specializes in floor dipping and chinning in various forms. Some variety is offered by dipping between two chairs as well as floor dipping. One hand dipping and one hand chinning are possible for the exceptional man who reaches that point. The movements described are not progressive, entirely too difficult for the heavy man; many big fellows, who are quite strong, can not chin even once. A man like Steve Stanko, bodyweight 220 pounds, who can chin with one hand is very, very exceptional. But he is the United States champion and made the highest two hands snatch and the highest clean and jerk of any of the world's lifters at the world's championships of Vienna last year. The light men find dipping and chinning too easy, too big a jump from the use of two hands to one. But some of them get there by making the exercise progressive by tying weights to the feet or laying them across the back in floor dipping. This form of exercise is better than no exercise, but it's so much easier to obtain much better results with progressive training with apparatus.

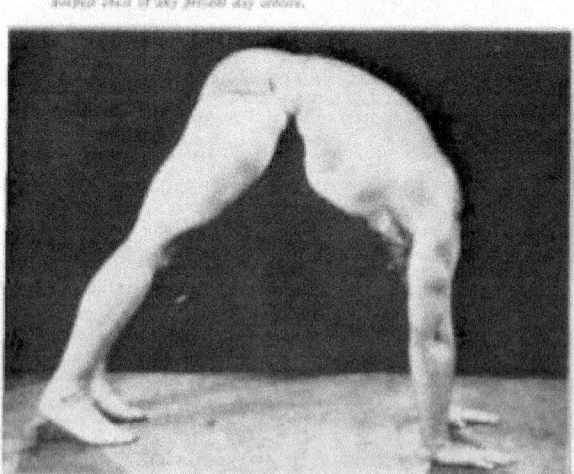

One of the Hindu Nomadic exercises as posed by Bob Hoffman. In this unretouched photo you can see why the author is believed to have the deepest chest of any present day athlete.

Some of the non-apparatus courses offer a variety of resistance exercises which employ imaginary resistance and, I must add, bring imaginary results. Yes, there is actually a course still being advertised which suggests that you pull on an imaginary rope and turn an imaginary wheel. Tensing exercises are recommended, exercises which would make the muscles of the man who already has them a bit more clear-cut, make possible additional control of the Biceps so that it can be displayed more prominently and thus gain a small fraction of an inch in apparent .size, but only in measurement. The same amount of effort placed back of real exercises would bring superior results.

When I wrote earlier in this chapter, what I formerly had constantly reiterated, that any exercise is better than no exercise, and now should qualify that oft-repeated statement, I had in mind resistance exercises, which resist one limb against another. These are more harmful than good. The reason seems to be that during the millions of generations which life has existed on this planet, the thousand or more generations during which man in his present form has been on this earth, certain habits of coordination have been developed. Only the men who had good coordination, who were so trained that the muscles would automatically do the right thing before being instructed by the brain, have survived. The survival of the fittest has brought men up to the present day, who with training are vastly superior in speed and athletic ability to any of the men of the past.

And as soon as you provide resistance for one part of the body with another, you break the laws of muscular movement which were developed in these many thousands of years. I am sure that this is the true answer. A great many men have reported a feeling of dizziness after practicing resisting one arm against the other for a time. They did not know why. And the reason is, that the brain which had been taught to direct the muscles along certain channels during all of human history becomes bewildered and mixed up with the muscular work that is being done. Resistance movements are not natural. And the worst of all of them is when there is an endeavor to provide resistance to one arm by using the other, such as in curling, or endeavoring to press.

Resistance may be applied in one or two ways without harm, such as the arms resisting the head for neck exercises, or the arms being held tight against each other in Pectoral development, or to tighten the muscles of the sides while rotating the body in a circular motion to develop the midsection.

To practice the several movements which I consider acceptable, not contrary to the many thousands of years of human training in coordination, you can proceed as follows: Place the hands, palms together, at about the height of the waist. Pressing hard together, keeping the hands close to the body, raise them to arm's length overhead. Relax for a moment. Then continuing to press bring them down and to the original position. There will be some beneficial action for the arms and you will feel the muscles of the chest flexing which of course will have a developmental effect. A similar movement can be practiced but one which brings the muscles into play in a somewhat different manner is as follows: Extend the arms down in front of the body, elbows straight, palms together, fingers locked. Keeping the arms straight, raise them to arm's length overhead, pressing them hard together throughout. Relax a moment, then pull hard as if endeavoring to separate them as the arms are brought down to the original position. In the first movement described, variation may be practiced in a similar manner while bringing the hands down.

Still another movement: Clasp the hands together keeping the arms bent and the hands close to the body; move them from side to side as far as possible in each direction resisting the push of one arm with the other. Vary this by pulling one arm with the other back and forth in a similar position. For the fourth resistance exercise: Extend the arms up directly overhead, straighten them and lock the fingers. Holding the arms and body tight, lean far to thr right, then far to the front, far to the left and lean well back. Continue this circular motion in such a manner that you can feel it in the muscles of the sides, back and abdomen. This movement will have some slight effect on the arms but is really a good mid-section exerciser.

If you are away, with no form of apparatus to use, you will obtain some small measure of benefit through the practice of non-apparatus movements, but if you really desire to build your strength and muscle (and you must or you wouldn't be reading this book) by all means put your efforts back of the proper training methods.

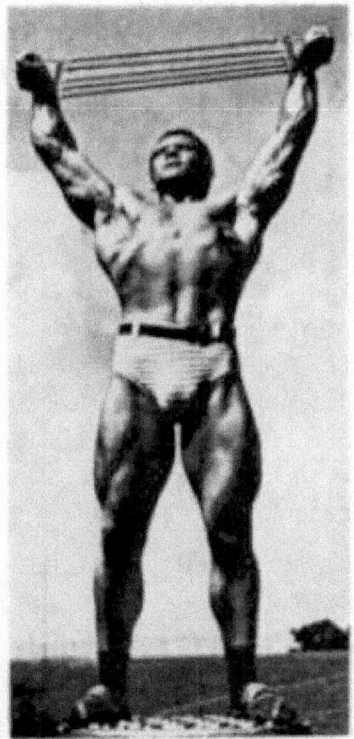

An exceptionally fine exercise picture of the popular muscular marvel, John Grimek.

Rope Climbing as a Means of Developing the Arm

IN the York bar bell gym there is a big rope suspended from the beam of the ceiling. Most of the York lifters at some time or other will take their turn at climbing that rope. All the star lifters are good rope climbers and the speed they make up that rope would compare favorably with the best of the champion rope climbers.

Considerable strength is required to climb a rope. I have seen men who had spent an important part of their training time at moderate physical training, curling and pressing with ten pound dumbells and working with a five cable exerciser with only moderate resistance, men who thought they were strong, who could not even climb a rope. By using the legs and the feet and pulling with both hands they would manage to get about half way up our rope. The exercises they practiced were so light that they could not handle their own bodyweight. Few untrained or partially trained men can hang by one hand on a rope. It takes a pretty fair grip. And few average humans could climb a rope if their lives depended upon it. If some dark night they fell from an anchored boat and then had to depend upon living by their ability to climb back up that rope to the deck, most of them would die in the process. Climbing a rope may save a life sometime and it is also the means of building strength and muscle.

While the untrained man or the fellow who uses moderate resistance, such as the methods most " train you by mail" instructors have advocated, can not even climb a rope, all the star lifters of the York team can climb a rope with their legs held at right angles from the body and with a considerable distance between each fresh hand grip. In coming down the rope, they come so exuberantly that each new hand grip is taken and then the entire body weight is pulled up and lowered. I feel certain that this moderate practice of rope climbing has added to the physical ability and lifting power of our strongest lifters.

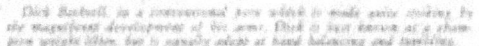

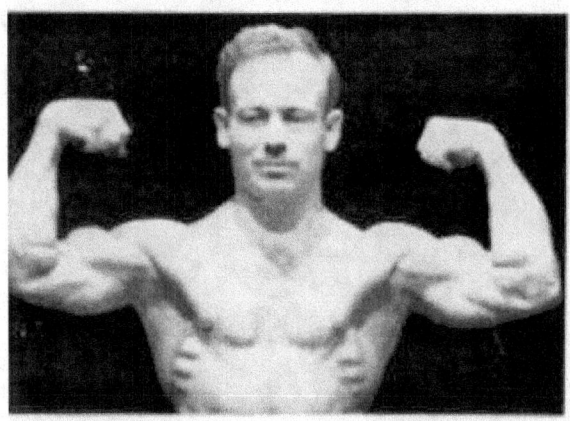

The act of hanging alone on a rope has a tendency to normalize the backbone if out of adjustment. It promotes the growth, increases the height, deepens the chest, makes the waist more muscular and slender, builds the Pectorals and shoulders as well as all parts of the arm. It brings into play the entire Biceps and the deeper lying Brachialis Amicus and Goracobrachialis.

If you find at the first attempt that you can not climb a rope you can start by pulling yourself from the floor with both hands. Then hold the rope with thighs and knees, with the calves and ankles if need be, while you reach up for a fresh two handed grip. Pull yourself up again, and continue as far as you can go. It will be slow and hard at first but you'll get there if you will persist. When you have climbed the rope, let yourself down hand over hand rather slowly, so thai your muscles will become strong enough that in time you can climb the rope hand over hand.

If you are tired when you reach the top, be careful not to come down so rapidly that you will burn or remove the skin from your palms. Make use of your knees and feet on the downward trip if the state of your strength demands. You'll strengthen in time through the persistent practice of this movement so that you can climb hand over hand and receive some added benefit from rope climbing.

The Arm Building Value of Giant Crushers and Iron Shoes

I HAVE always enjoyed the use of the giant crusher grip. It is popular with most body culturists who like to vary their training by an occasional session with an appliance that permits a different arm movement with resulting development from a different angle.

Years ago I obtained one of the curved springs which Breitbart offered with his course of training. It consisted of a number of steel leaves or springs, and was made somewhat like a miniature automobile spring. Its chief objection was the fact that the steel leaves would break at times with possible damage to the user. Several lawsuits were pending when the company gave up its manufacture and sale. But I enjoyed using mine. About 1925 I carried with me in my travels, which consisted of about fifty thousand miles a year via Model T Ford, one of these Breitbart springs, a ten cable set and a 105 pound bar bell. I would chase prospects or " suspects " all day long, write a letter home to my firm and then spend an hour or two with the appliances I carried with me. It worked well too, for without any other training I managed to enter and have fair success in any athletic competition I could find on Saturday in or near the cities where I happened to be. I had made the particular trip about which I am now writing through Pittsburgh, Erie, Toledo, Cleveland, Detroit, Fort Wayne and then back to Pittsburgh again. I won 44 medals on that trip in a variety of events, principally aquatics, which was my specialty, canoeing, rowing and swimming. But I also entered a boxing contest, a shot putting contest and the broad jump at a track and field meet. I am sure that the crusher grip aided my development and helped me acquire these forty-four medals which I brought home. I realize too that the cables and particularly the bar bell brought even better results, but all were means to the end of improving my endurance, speed, skill, strength and development.

Today we have only the hand crusher and the giant crusher grip to offer. The hand crusher is made progressive because it is made in three strengths. Two grips can be used in one hand later and reasonable progression is possible. It provides one of the best known means of developing the grip. The Giant Crusher is not progressive, but it provides such stiff resistance that it can not be bent by the beginner in some ways. Only after considerable training is this possible and then really good all around results will be obtained. Cables can not provide resistance for the crushing muscles of the body. Dumbell exercises while lying on boxes or a bench will at least partially simulate the movement of the crusher grip, but not entirely. The crusher provides greatest resistance when nearly closed, just at the point where dumbells have ceased to offer resistance as they are held overhead. I believe a crusher grip should be part of the training equipment of every really ambitious body culturist.

Then there is the device best known as the German Iron Shoe. As you can see from the illustration it is not unlike a giant horseshoe. It brings the muscles into play in an exactly opposite manner to the Giant Crusher Grip. At one time I read a letter from a man who actually claimed to have increased the size of his arm six full inches through the use of the Iron Shoe. I can't believe that, for a device such as the Iron Shoe does not provide sufficient range of movement to develop so huge an arm. There are men who will say anything to win a prize for the best physical improvement as occasionally offered by the people who sell a course of physical training. A big cup is often offered for the greatest gains in a certain period of training and I am sorry to say that often the biggest tall talc teller wins.

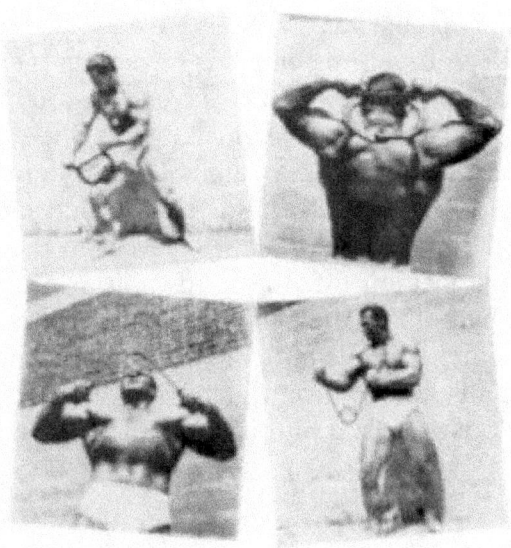

The Iron Shoe will greatly strengthen the pulling and tearing muscles of the hands, arms and shoulders. It operates the muscles from a different angle again and will make it possible to apply one's strength in diverse manners. There is no way in which quite the same action can be had with weights or even with cables, which do work in a slightly similar manner. The Iron Shoe is especially good for the fellow who wishes to add to his strength reputation by bending spikes, breaking chains, tearing decks of cards or telephone books, bending bottle tops, or even bending worn-out horseshoes. There are men who have broken horseshoes, but I am quite confident that there has never been a man who could bend and break a new, never before handled horseshoe. Try this sometime and see if you agree with me.

Iron Shoe training will give you hands like a vise, will greatly strengthen the tendons and ligaments and will develop powerful corded muscles of hands, arms and shoulders. The exerciser can be made progressive by using

135

additional springs and stronger springs. There is a certain amount of wear and tear, breaking and weakening of the springs with an Iron Shoe which is never present with dumbells, although sets of springs have withstood a year of continuous work. You can hold the Iron Shoe directly in front of you and pull it apart with both arms doing an equal share of the work. You can hold it to the side and, keeping first the right arm straight, pull it apart with the left. Then reverse the position of the arms. You can vary the movement by holding the hand grips of the exerciser down and up at other times; you can pull it while leaning with one handle of the exerciser against the ground. You may hold it back of neck and pull it out in that entirely different position.

When I was a member of a championship rowing crew in 1926 I kept my cables and spring exerciser in my locker and had a lot of fun trying out the fellows who thought they were strong at bending and stretching my appliances. The muscles have the happy faculty of becoming accustomed to the movement they are asked to perform very quickly. Therefore a man who has done some cable, crushei or Iron Shoe work can easily outdo an even stronger man who has never had the advantage of this special training.

You'll have a lot of fun with these appliances; you'll develop strength and muscle and travel farther on the road to the acquisition of the biggest, best developed and most powerful arm that is possible for your bony framework and bodyweight.

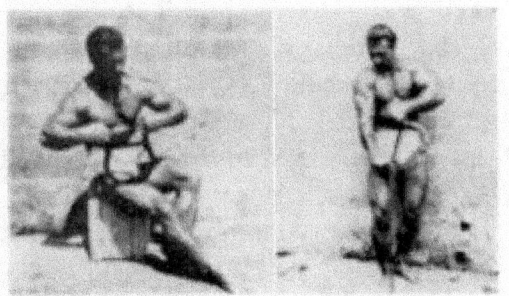

John Grewet exercising with the Iron Shoe.

Cables in Arm Development

CABLES are used universally; more in England and European countries, I believe, than in America, for over there it has long been the practice to hold cable pulling championships. There have been some men with magnificently developed arms who made a specialty of cable stretching and the winning of these contests. While cables are best known as a means of developing the shoulders, upper arms and chest they provide a great deal of resistance for the Triceps in particular. The stirrups, which are a part of the York Home Gym, make possible the practice of most of the dumbell exercises which have brought such good results—the front curl, back curl, upright rowing motion and of course the various forms of pressing.

Years ago there was a strong man from the Argentine, Belvidere Del Monte by name, who had developed a pair of wonderful arms, principally through the use of expanders. Not more than a half dozen men in the world, it is believed, could stretch his expanders. He concentrated so much on arm development and cable pulling strength, neglecting his lower body, that he had only a 21 1/2 inch thigh—not much larger than a really strong man's arm. He had only mediocre ability at handling weights because the largest and most powerful muscles of the body—the legs and lower back— had been neglected.

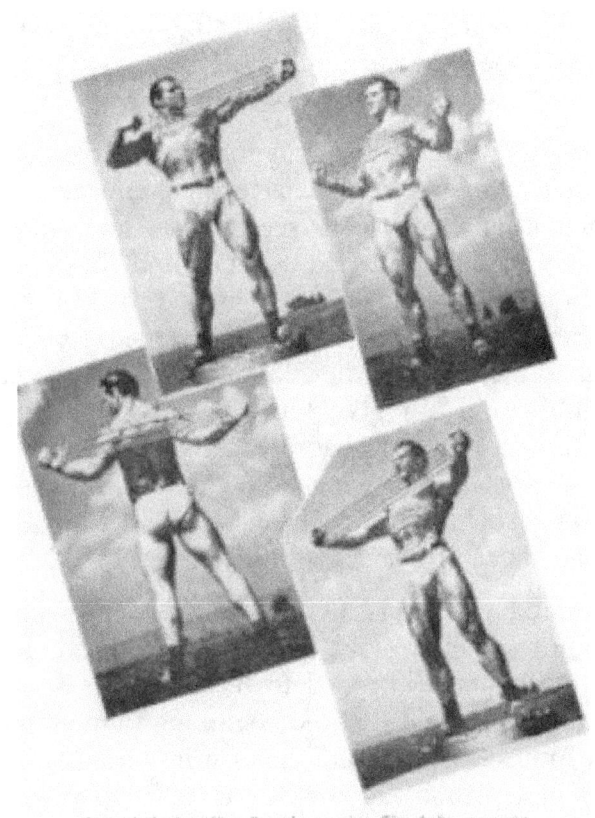

Some of the best Chest Expander exercises, The Archer movement, Front Press, Back Press and the Chest Pull. Need we tell you that John Grimek has posed for these exercises?

Seguinel, a famous European expander specialist, has a simply wonderful Triceps and his entire upper body development is exceptional. He like Del Monte does not have the strength to handle heavy weights. Joseph Vanderznaden, known as the " strong Belgian," was perhaps the strongest expander puller of his day. Even the famous French authority, Prof. Desbonnet, considered Vanderznaden's arm to rank among the best. There is a good reason for this, however, for aside from his proficiency at cable pulling he also trained almost daily with weights. He not only had huge arms, but really strong ones too, through this all around training, and was capable of a great many strength feats besides cable pulling.

Fred Rollon was considered by a great many European authorities to be the most magnificently developed man who existed in their time. He had a most unusual muscular development and muscular separation—was, in fact, a human anatomical chart. He concentrated for years upon cable training and became the recognized world's champion of the cable pulling art. Cables accounted for the truly remarkable upper body development he possessed. His cable pulling did not give him the ability to lift heavy weights and he was so chagrined at times through being bested by smaller men, with not nearly his impressive development, that he took up the regular practice of weight training and became a successful lifter.

There are certain exercises which can be done with cables that are not possible or as convenient with weights. Although this book is intended to be a treatise on arm development, we promised at the beginning to mention allied groups of muscles which aid the arm in doing its intended work. The Latissimus Dorsi is one of these groups and this muscle can best be developed with cables. As explained in the chapter on anatomy, its purpose is to pull the arms down from overhead. There is no way that this can be done with weights, for weights are heavy and must be pushed or jerked overhead and held there. They come down fast enough of themselves through the force of gravity without the possibility of pulling them down. Therefore the exercise in which the arms are held at full length overhead, being held straight throughout and then pulled down to shoulder height, not only strengthens and develops the Latissimus better than any other exercise, but also assists in the development of the upper arm muscles which attach to the Trapezius, the tendons too, and of course accounts for considerable development of the upper arm.

Another exercise which is possible with cables and can not be practiced with dumbells, one that develops the arms and shoulders from a somewhat different angle, is the pull to straight arms at shoulder height with cables. The arms are extended to the front, at shoulder height, and then holding them straight are pulled until they are fully extended at the sides. This is primarily a good Deltoid developer, but the arms must withstand considerable of the effort of stretching the cable and of course as in the previous exercise receive considerable development.

The archer's movement is one of the popular cable exercises not possible with dumbells. One arm is extended to the side at full length and shoulder height. The other with the knuckles front is pulled away, just like pulling the string of a bow except that it is extended to full length in the opposite direction. The hands should be reversed in practicing this exercise. Pressing both arms simultaneously with the hands held in front of the body brings the arms and shoulders into action in a different manner than does any weight exercise. The hark press is one of the very best for developing the Triceps, Deltoids, and the side or bent pressing ability. Although a similar movement can be practiced with dumbells, an exercise that many consider the best Triceps developer known to physical training, it's wise to practice it at times with cables. It's this movement more than any other which has developed the really remarkable arms of some star cable pullers. For in this style greater resistance can be overcome, more strands stretched than in any other way.

If you were to travel through Europe you could not find a department or sporting goods store without cables. Nor could you find any sort of gymnasium, where a group of men train, without their cables. When we went to Germany to the Olympics in 1936, we saw cables everywhere. Made of steel and some of the most tremendous rubber strands anyone could imagine, it would take a real strong man to progressively move from one to another in the various exercises. The majority of the great German lifters, the men who hold the championships, European and world's records, incorporate considerable of cable training with their weight lifting practice. When the German team came here to meet our strong men in an international team match to determine the world's championship weight lifting team, each brought a set of cables with them. These were used in addition to the weight lifting training while here, but served as the sole training medium while on the sea and traveling from place to place where weights were not always available.

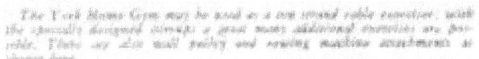

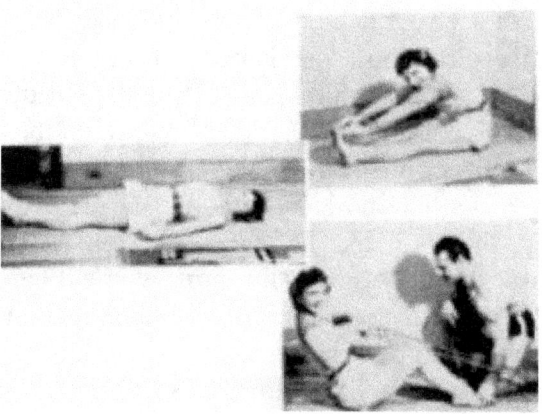

The best physiques in the world have the indelible stamp of cable training upon them. The multitude of movements possible with a modern cable set build strength and muscle from every angle, more muscles are brought into play and a superior shapeliness and greater strength result. Cables are invaluable for the man who is unable to use weights at home, owing perhaps to limited space, the fact that he lives in a furnished room or apartment where others would be bothered by even the slight sound of weight training. Or perhaps he is a man who can make one or two visits weekly to a Y. M. C. A. or gymnasium where weights arc available. This is not enough to more than keep a man in condition. To make progress there should be not less than three training periods weekly, preferably four, and for the man who does not perform physical labor of any sort, five training periods will be best if he is really ambitious.

Cables will keep the muscles in condition on the intervening days when it is not possible to visit the gymnasium and handle heavy weights. Cables will "tone the muscles," as Rudi Ismayr, the German weight lifting captain, Olympic champion of 1932, world champion other years, had to say in explanation of the use of cables by the members of his team as well as himself. Cable training prepares the muscles for the harder work to come where heavy weights are employed. All men who strive for great strength, weight lifting ability, a perfect physique with really big arms, should use cables.

Cables serve best in developing the muscles which are so conspicuous in the male physique. They impart a certain shapeliness to the physique which can not be acquired in any other way. They build magnificent shoulders, well muscled, rounded, heavily muscled chests, a fine development of the upper back and powerful, admiration creating arms.

At lifting shows, weight lifting clinics, conventions of physical directors and other gatherings where men interested in the development of the human body will gather, I am frequently asked if our strong men use cables. Did John Grimek use cables? The answer is yes, and it would be yes if you asked about many other forms of training. For like all men who obtain the ultimate in strength and development, Grimek has spent considerable time with cables. And he also has done most everything else in the line of lifting, bar bell and dumbell work, balancing and all sorts of manly physical activities and games. For I do not know of one really outstanding physique which is not the result of the " thousand exercises." It takes all around training to bring out the strength and the greatest possibilities of the muscles in shapeliness. While I am on the subject 1 perhaps had better explain what the " thousand exercises" means. Many have written in to inquire. It means only that the men have performed a thousand different body building exercises—all they can think of or learn about.

Some of the finest built men in the world have devoted a great deal of their training time to cable training. In looking over photos of an old catalogue showing men who had gained strength and development through cables, we see the photo of Kenneth Terrill, one of the finest built men ever developed in this country. Gregory Paradise, one of the most powerful of the smaller men, a man who chins repeatedly with one finger. And Charles Atlas of " train you by mail without apparatus " fame. Yes, he was a star cable pupil; his photo appears in the catalogue, and cables helped him to the physique which has made his life so much easier and more profitable. It would be interesting not just to compile a list of the strength and development stars of the day who have used cables, but of the few who have not used them—hardly a man who has not used cables at some stage of his career.

While cables bring best results for the upper arm in all sorts of pressing and stretching movements, there are a number of good exercises for the front of the arm. One and two hand curling can be practiced with the stirrups and one hand curling by thrusting one foot through the handle of the cable set. Lateral and forward raise, upright rowing motion, spreading the arms to the side while leaning; back hand curl and many other movements greatly assist in the building and strengthening of the arm.

Hand Balancers Have Big Arms

IF you have regularly attended vaudeville theatres you must have seen many men who perform a hand to hand act who have magnificent upper arm development. You have observed their routine and you must have noted that they perform a great many Herculean feats. The top mounter not only must retain a balance in many difficult positions, but frequently must pull himself up and press out to the hand stand position. In this movement he is first curling and then pressing his bodyweight and it is natural that he should obtain favorable results from the practice and performance of such movements. The top mounter may perform a one hand stand, which of course provides even more vigorous movement for the arm.

The understander at all times must support the weight of his partner, in addition to pressing him out in a variety of ways in the progress of the act. Men who are star performers in Herculean hand to hand balancing have tremendous developments. Otto Arco and brother, and at one time Emile Margorissey, performed such an act, and Otto who did the understanding had one of the finest developments which ever graced a human being. We must remember that he had been a weight lifter, was one of the first three men in the history of the world to elevate double his bodyweight overhead. Bert Goodrich, a man who has flashed across the physical culture world particularly in the last few years and been the winner of a number of physical excellence awards and Mr. America contests, is also an understander in a hand to hand act. But he has been a tumbler, ring and horizontal bar performer, shot putter, discus thrower and javeline thrower, sprinter, stunt man of the movies and has trained with bar bells for many years. Bar bells, so he says, brought him to the point where he can now perform some of his most sensational feats which were not possible without the special weight training.

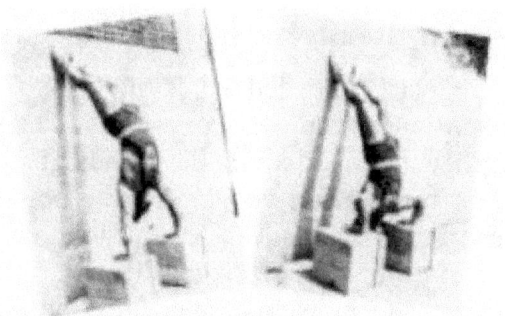

Just plain hand balancing is of little benefit in developing the upper arms. Kicking up into a balance requires practically no exertion of the upper arm. You must have seen small boys and girls and frail ladies who could hand balance yet had no noticeable development of the upper arm. In such balancing the body is supported by a column of bone. Movement is necessary to develop muscles. The best results are obtained when the muscle operates over its entire range, from extreme contraction to extreme extension.

It is a tremendously big step from the usual kick up or throw up into the hand stand, to the point where you can push up into a hand stand. Development can be obtained by pushing into a hand stand. Most of the men who have been among the leaders in perfect man contests practice some balancing. It provides more of the "thousand exercises " which result in the best physiques. It produces a certain amount of all round development, balance, coordination, physical skill, especially if some tumbling movements are practiced with other exercises. But the real results from a development standpoint obtained by the hand balancer come from performing dips in the hand stand position and from press ups and tiger bends. The first exercise is usually performed with feet against the wall, so that it becomes a muscle developing exercise, not just a balancing feat. Pressing with the hands on two boxes permits a greater range of movement and has added to the pressing ability of most of the champion lifters.

Men who already have at least a fair amount of strength may learn to hand balance by pushing into the hand stand position. To learn this movement the hands are placed in their position usually about shoulder width apart with the fingers parallel and pointing to the front. The knees are placed outside the straight elbows.

The Biceps receives little benefit from balancing. But the Triceps which, as mentioned several times before, forming as it does about two-thirds of the bulk of the upper arm, will gain in size and strength and result in larger arm size.

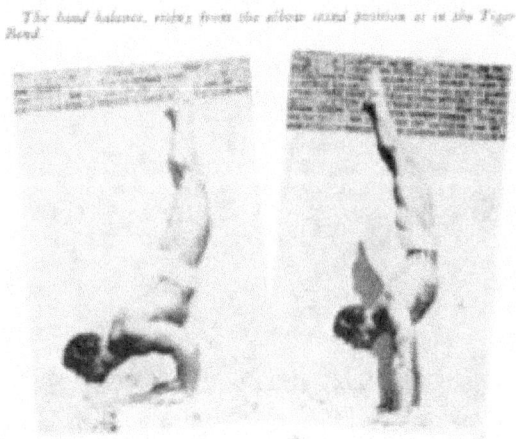

The hand balance, rising from the elbow stand position as in the Tiger Bend.

The tiger bend is a feat only possible to an advanced weight frian and balancer. The very best performers are capable of a dozen or more consecutive bends. This consists of lowering to the elbow balance position, then with a forward lean and an upward thrust of the legs the balancing position with straight arms is regained. Continue to lower and raise as long as possible. It's hard work. Hard work is required to develop a lot of muscle. Exercise itself is easy enough, but there is one rule we must remember concerning physical training. We obtain from exercise what we put into it. Train moderately easily and you receive moderate results. Train vigorously, to the limit of your strength and endurance, at times and you receive results in direct proportion to the effort put forth.

Dumbell Training

I HAVE been hurrying through the other forms of body building, especially of arm building, with and without apparatus of other sorts for I have been anxious to get down to the real means of training—to weights, especially of the little short-handled bells, dumbells.

Bar bells antedate dumbells in physical training. Bar bells, simply a long-handled dumbell, permitting its use with two hands, have been in use for thousands of years. In cities and towns in the distant interior of China, where they hardly know of the existence of the remainder of the world or even of the war that is in progress, there are groups of bar bells, frequently in the center of the village or hamlet where the youth of the town come to train, build their strength and prove their manhood. These bar bells consist of stones of various sizes through which a shaft has been thrust. The weaker men start with the lighter weights, the stronger men progress up to the heaviest, gaining increasing renown as they become strong enough to reach the heights.

It is said that Japan copied practically everything from their bigger and formerly more progressive neighbor, China. Bar bells travelled from China to Japan, for the smart little people of Nippon are quick to recognize and to copy any system superior to their own. Many photos wrrc published of physical training in Japan which show the great athletes of that nation training with bar bells, stone bar bells, better constructed than the Chinese bar bells. The stones are nice appearing products of the stone cutter's art, somewhat similar to small millstones of a century or so ago, but thicker and smaller in diameter. Made in various sizes and weights the same sort of training is possible which was the rule in this country a half century ago prior to the advent of the plate loading bar bell which made training more progressive.

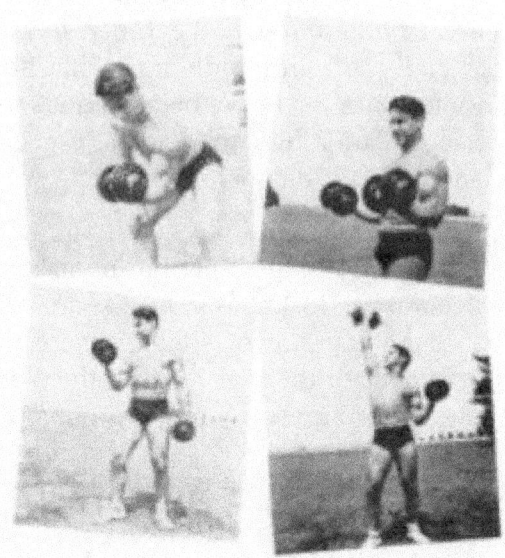

During these years a great many men lifted stones, sometimes one large stone, but frequently a stone in each hand. They could easily discover the much greater possibilities of exercises with a weight in each hand, the much greater range of movement. But it was not until the 16th century, just four hundred years ago, that the first dumbells of which we have a record appeared. They were found in England, and were called dumbells because they bore some resemblance to a bell, but having no clapper were dumb. From that time on, they travelled around the world and were adopted with most enthusiasm in continental Europe.

The great strong men of fifty years ago, in particular, were the product of very heavy dumbell training to a considerable degree. Very heavy dumbells are hard to handle. While Joseph Manger, world's and Olympic champion at present, holder of the two hands press record at 317 pounds, a man who has jerked 410 pounds, is very powerful, he had great difficulty in cleaning or pulling to the shoulders in one movement a pair of hundred pound dumbells. It required five attempts before he got them there. Then it was absurdly easy for him to press them overhead. I talked to George Hackenschmidt on his recent visit to this country. He was a Russian, former world's lifting and wrestling champion. He was at his best in 1908. He told me of a trip that he made to Vienna to engage in a weight lifting contest. He had never lifted heavy dumbells, only using them as an exercising medium, so had great difficulty in getting heavy dumbells to the shoulder—additional proof that heavy dumbell lifting will bring great results in developing muscle.

I am a great believer in dumbell training. I like to train with them myself and have urged, usually with success, all the lifters with whom I come into contact to use dumbells in their training. While in England, a number of their 42 official lifts are done with dumbells. In my recent book on " Weight Lifting," I did not include any lift with two dumbells, such as the two dumbells clean and jerk, or the continental and press with two dumbells or the two dumbell swing. My book includes one dumbell swing, bent press, side press and military press in which dumbells may be used, but not the heavy dumbell lifting the old timers used. There are so many exercises and I believe that dumbells lend themselves better as a means of training rather than as a means of establishing lifting records.

I haven't been able to explain it, but when I started my professional career, teaching bar bell and dumbell training and writing books and articles upon the subject, a real furore was created when people of certain quarters found that I was advocating dumbell training. In fact such an issue was made about it, that for a time it seemed that the weight training world of America would be divided against itself. It was a bit ridiculous, but one of the leading writers on the subject, who was constantly advocating overemphasis on deep knee bending and dead lifting, the handling of the heaviest possible weights, thought or at least told the world that dumbells would make you slow and muscle bound while the heavier lifting wouldn't. Now that was ridiculous. Of course there is no such thing as muscle bound as the result of lifting weights. But one thing sure, moderate dumbell training would not result in such an effect if the heaviest of bar bell lifting would not.

As time went on and we included a pair of dumbells with our bar bell set, instead of the kettle bells and single dumbell handle offered by our competitors, people quickly found that the system of training I was advocating brought best results. In two and a half short years from the time we issued our first Strength and Health Magazine, the other people went bankrupt and we bought them out. Their principal instructor has tried to start again on several occasions, and has admitted that we were right by offering a pair of dumbells with his weight training set.

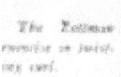 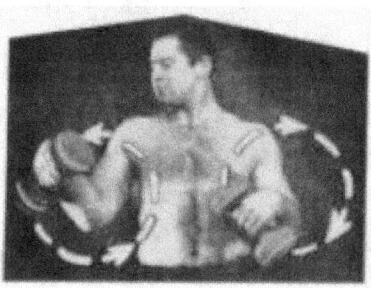

The Roseman exercise on instructing curl.

We were right in the beginning in believing that dumbells were a very important part of physical training and now the entire weight training world believes as we do. My system of weight training revolutionized the physical training world and my training methods are universally used.

Dumbells never wear out. They offer equal resistance every inch of the way. Unlike cables which are easy at the start of the movement and more difficult as the movement progresses and the cable stretches to near its limit, dumbells always offer the same resistance. While any form of equipment that relies for its resistance upon springs or rubber will weaken in time, dumbells and of course their partner, bar bells, may be handed down from father to son and from grandfather to grandson. They never wear out— can be used by an entire family—the young people, girls and boys, father and mother, the old folks too.

With dumbells there are three best exercises: The one hand curl to develop the front of the arm, the side press to develop the back of the arm, and the upright rowing motion. You could obtain a marvelous arm by practicing these three movements either singly, with either one hand or two; or as a compound exercise. In the first sentence of this paragraph I mentioned that the one hand curl and the side press were two of the three best. In practicing with one hand at a time, you can concentrate upon the development of that single arm. Then instead of resting between movements as you must do with two hand exercises, you can just change hands and go on with exercising the other arm, then come back to the first arm, etc.

I have said little enough about compound exercises. They have unusual merit. While it is not good training to select a weight light enough that more than fifteen movements are possible, with compound exercises you can perform thirty to fifty, depending upon whether three or five exercises, ten movements each, are practiced in series. You can perform thirty to fifty movements in this manner for the changed movement of the arms serves as a partial rest between exercises. During your next training period, take a pair of dumbells. You should select the most weight which will permit you to practice ten properly executed curls. The curl, as we have mentioned on several occasions, will develop the Biceps, the upright rowing motion the Brach- ialis Anticus and to a fair degree the Coracobrachialis. This comes very close to being my favorite exercise. I know it is my favorite dumbell exercise and rivals the bent press and the two hands snatch as my all around favorites. This exercise will build muscle, pulling power and all around strength. Before my annual birthday contest of 1937, I took a pair of forty pound dumbells with me to the annual A. A. U. meeting in Boston. There I specialized on this exercise—was successful upon my return in officially snatching 230 pounds, which bettered my own lifetime record by ten pounds. This movement develops the arm, the shoulders and the Trapezius muscles—the muscle group which imparts the pleasing slope to the shoulders.

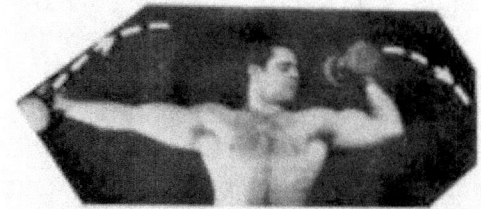

Steve Stanko, performing the alternate curl at shoulder height.

Pinaski Vaclav, one of the best heavyweight lifters of the present. He was runner up to hold the Olympics of 1932 and 1936. He presses 286 pounds, weighs 233 at his height of five feet four, and possesses 18¼ inch arms.

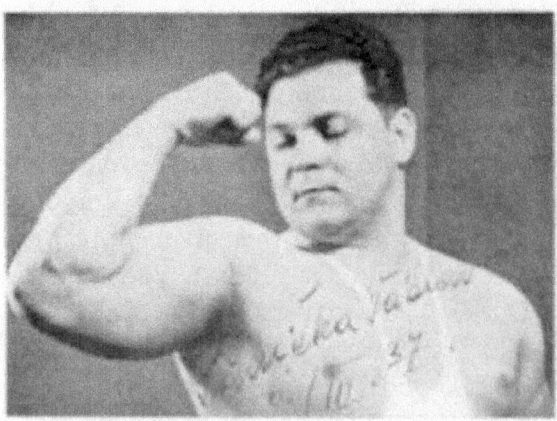

Ten curls, ten upright rowing motions and then you can perform the side press simultaneously with each arm. This exercise is normally practiced with a single arm and is a marvelous developer of the Deltoids, the Triceps and the

Latissimus, but it can be practiced in this series with a dumbell in each hand. This compound exercise practiced with three outstanding movements could be repeated each training session or several times a training session and bring very good results.

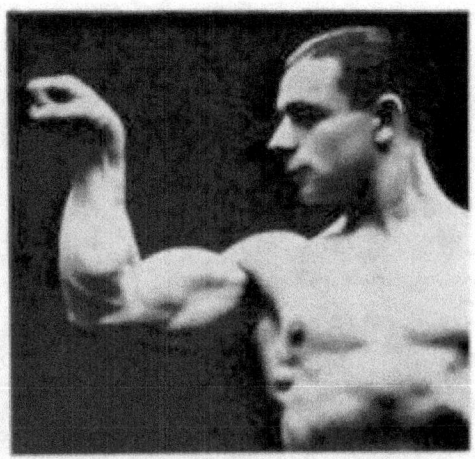

While this particular pose of Siegmund Klein does not show the biceps to its greatest advantage, it does depict large arm size and splendid forearm development.

With dumbells you have three basic movements, and scores of variations of these movements. Three movements are curl, pull and press. With the curl there is the front curl, the back curl, the curl with thumbs up, the twisting curl, made popular or famous by the great old timer George Zottman. These exercises are normally performed standing erect. They can be done with single arm, both arms simultaneously or alternately. They bring good results if performed while leaning forward. There is a temptation in curling with one or two arms to rest the elbow against the body, thus using it as a center for leverage. This is not possible when leaning over; the exercise is purely muscular and good results are sure to be obtained.

While these movements, leaning, can be practiced with both hands together, I prefer to rest one hand upon a low box to support the weight of the body and then perform the

155

front and back curl and the rowing motion. Never fail to exercise the other arm.

Of the men who have been renowned for their muscles, Eugene Sandow leads the list. Although he used bar bells as well as dumbells, it is evident that the greater portion of his time was placed back of dumbell training. His one arm press record of 271 pounds was greater than his two hands clean and jerk record of 250. His record in the one hand clean and jerk, from all that I can find in perusing the old books, was 165 pounds. He claimed a phenomenal record in the one hand military press, a record which exceeded the 125 pounds credited to Arthur Saxon, a man who exceeded his bent press record by a full hundred pounds, but I fear that we will have to relegate this great military press record to a figment of the imagination of one of his press agents as we must do with his normal 16 1/2 inch arm which somehow or other grew in the reports to a huge 19 inch extremity.

Nevertheless, it would be difficult to find a more perfectly moulded arm than Sandow's. His wrist was small in comparison which made the upper arm especially huge looking. Sandow, particularly in his earlier career, before he let the' desire to make a few more dollars enter into his sale of the light " gadget," the spring dumbell of three and five pounds, was free to tell the world that weights, principally dumbell training, were solely responsible for his great development. He explained that when he was young, he was a mere stripling, thinner than the average and rather frail and that weights were solely responsible for the physique which won for him undying fame.

Another factor in Sandow's favor—he was thin skinned. Although John Grimek feels that he is not thin skinned, the fact does remain that the combination of extraordinary development, and skin thinner than other big men, has made a physique for him which permits every muscle to be seen to the greatest detail. Either Grimek or Sandow had and have marvelous muscles, but if they had been cloaked with thicker skin they would not have been nearly so nice in appearance.

In this world of ours, it has been proven that no one man can have everything. Sandow was handsome of face and figure, had beautiful curly hair and an attractive little mustache, was a great favorite everywhere, all of which won for him acclaim and the love of a most beautiful wife, but he did not have the great strength of some men who do not have his proportions and muscular definition. The smooth muscles which are not nearly so evident are much stronger than the more finely drawn muscles. One need only consider the muscles of Arthur Saxon as they appeared in the photos we have, or the arm of Manger, the world's champion, or Psenicka who made the second highest press of the world's lifters, or the huge arms of Stanko and Dave Mayor. The first two arms mentioned are quite smooth, the second two not really smooth, but not as thin skinned as Sandow's.

It's desirable for the body builder to strive for an arm like Sandow's. But if you don't get the same type of arm, don't be disappointed. For the stronger the arm, the more dense the bundles of tiny muscular fibres, and the smoother should be the arm. You will be able to build a fine arm if you persist, and if you don't get an arm exactly of the shape of Sandow's, you will find that nature has compensated you by giving thicker tendons, and thicker muscle groups.

In beginning to practice the two hands curl, unless you who read this are very weak, you will find thirty pounds in two hands curling sufficiently heavy to begin. The handle should be about shoulder width apart and the bar evenly balanced. The hands are held at arm's length at the start of the movement, turned slightly back against the body and the elbows straight. From this position the wrists should be bent and kept bent throughout the movement as this adds to the development of the forearm. The movement is continued with fair slowness until the bell reaches the shoulders. You should be careful that you do not swing or jerk the weight to the chest. Then lower it slowly, so that you can feel the weight in the Biceps as it is lowered. With the elbows kept close to the sides and the curling done slowly with the power of the arms, better results will be obtained.

After you have passed the double progressive stage of starting as low as five, try to continue with a weight you can handle ten times. After performing the movement ten times for a few exercise periods, try eleven, and then twelve, finally work up to fifteen, then increase the poundage and start again at ten.

 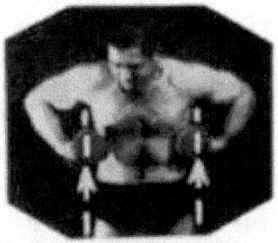

You should not fail to practice the reverse curl. And be sure that you have the dumbells turned so that the knuckles are directly up. It is so easy to let the weights swing to a point where the thumb is straight up.

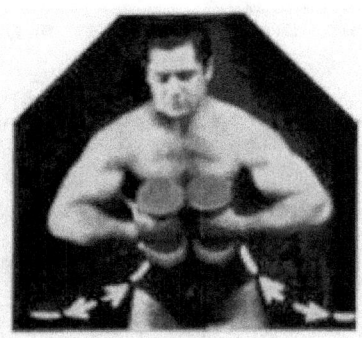

This would be exercise No. 102, in it is not included in the 101 dumbell exercises. The dumbells are curled from a position well out from the body to the position shown here.

One arm curling is included among the lifts in my book, " Weight Lifting." So we can look forward to some curling contests and some really fine records being established. At present I do not know of anyone who has curled in correct style 200 pounds. There are men who can curl a hundred pounds; a great many who can curl seventy-five pounds. In fact men as powerful as John Grimek and John Davis could exercise with a 75 pound bell in each hand. Horace Barre was given credit for having curled a 100 pound dumbell three times in succession. But he was a huge man, weighing all of 300 pounds, a good part of it muscle. Louis Cyr was given credit for having performed a one hand curl of over 200 pounds. But this sounds like entirely too much. If he performed a one hand curl with the assistance of the other and the elbow resting on the thigh, he probably could have curled a great deal of weight, for I saw Siegmund Klein curl the Cyr dumbell weighing 202 pounds to his shoulder and bent press it at a York strength show several years ago. Many men can muscle out more than they can curl. Muscling out is practiced more frequently than curling for it is not believed that the front curl has any really beneficial effect on developing lifting ability and the strong men I know best are lifters. Therefore they do not practice the two hands curl. But I have seen John Davis, world's 181 pound champion, when requested, perform successive and correct two hand curls with 150 pounds.

We will now turn our attention to the Triceps or back of the upper arm group. Any work done or any lifting movement where a weight, heavy or light, is pushed or lifted above the head and shoulders will more or less develop the back of the arm. But as well regulated, methodical, systematic, intelligently and progressively arranged exercises alone will bring the best, quickest and surest results, a few of the most effective Triceps exercises with dumbells will be described. The exercises which are well known as shoulder developers in many cases are equally fine for building the upper arms—especially the one arm side press, bent press, or the two hands military press.

One of my three best dumbell exercises for developing the arm is the side press. This can be started by the body builder with little experience with 25 pounds. Fifty pounds is easy enough for the more advanced lifter, while 75 to 100 pounds are within the capacity of the real lifter. This is a lift in which it is wise to progress slowly. Confine yourself to the starting poundage for four to six weeks. Then increase only five pounds. And after another four week period change again. Trying to hurry too fast will result in making a lift, rather than an exercise, of the movement and undersized, stringy arms may be the result instead of the bulging, rounded, powerful arms so much to be desired.

In the side press it is highly important that the correct position be assumed. When using the right arm, stand with the right foot pointing straight ahead, the left foot about twenty-four inches to the side and pointing off at an angle. This position of the feet is reversed when the left arm is used. The athlete picks up the dumbell and holds it in position at shoulder height so that the dumbell is not pointing straight to the front, but on a line parallel with the shoulders. The free arm is held out straight from the side at shoulder height. With moderate slowness the weight should then be pressed or pushed up to arm's length above the head, the body leaned toward the side away from the lifting arm. As he leans over, the free hand should touch the side of the leg near the knee. The weight should then be lowered slowly, straightening the body as the original or starting position is regained. As the bell is lowered it must be stopped before it comes down to the point of touching the shoulder—a bit to the rear, but not much lower than the shoulder. This exercise may be practiced as few as five or six times in the very beginning, but work up to ten as soon as you can. When you reach the point of handling substantial poundages, you can use the system of three times five groups of repetitions.

If a man works up to seventy-five or eighty pounds in this exercise, and can perform as many as twenty movements to test himself some training day, he will then have a really powerful and well-developed Triceps.

Another good Triceps exercise is practiced with two dumbells of moderate weight. Lean forward so that the body is inclined at right angles to the legs. Holding the knuckles up, upper arms in line with the back, alternately straighten and bend the arms. You will quickly feel the results of this movement in the ache your Triceps experiences.

There are numberless good arm exercises, most of which I intend to enumerate later, but I want you to remember that you can get all the arm that any man would want, a pair of arms, with Triceps and Biceps which will possess classical contours, that will symbolize great power and strength if you will practice just the two hands curl in its various forms, the side press, military press with dumbells, bent press, alternate press; in briefer words, a variety of curling and pressing movements with the addition of a little upright and bent over rowing.

Developing The Arms With The Bar Bell

THE bar bell permits the use of two hands with each exercise and a much heavier poundage can be employed. The basic exercises practiced with the bar bell have been at least partially described in the treatise on dumbell training. Curl, rowing and press are the possible movements. The two hands curl with bar bell is the most regularly practiced Biceps developer with bar bell. It should be practiced as I described in the dumbell curl, from extreme contraction to extreme extension. Slowly curl or pull the weight from its position across the thighs, until it touches the upper part of the chest. Continue this movement for the specified number of counts on each exercise day—heavy and light on your limit day of training, up to fifteen on one training day—and select a poundage you can lift ten times on the other major training day.

The reverse curl is commonly practiced although it develops the Biceps but little. But it does provide a roundness of development for the Biceps which is very pleasing to behold. The Brachioradialis is the muscle which receives the greatest benefit from this particular movement. By all means include this exercise in your training and perform it correctly. It is so easy to execute a back hand swing or to permit the elbows to leave the sides as you perform a combination rowing motion and curl. Employ the weight which permits you to correctly perform this exercise with the elbows held against the sides.

The rowing motion is most commonly practiced leaning over with the upper body parallel to the floor. A good poundage can be handled in this exercise. At times if you are interested in becoming a star weight lifter, it is permissible to handle a weight so heavy that it must be pulled to the chest with a motion and help of the upper body. But as a general thing it is better to select a weight which permits correct performance of this movement. You can rest your head upon a chair to be sure that you don't raise it during the progress of the exercise. The rowing motion can be practiced with the hands very wide apart, and the elbows out, and for variety and to develop the pulling muscles from a different angle, space the hands shoulder width apart and pull the weight to the body with the elbows turned toward the sides.

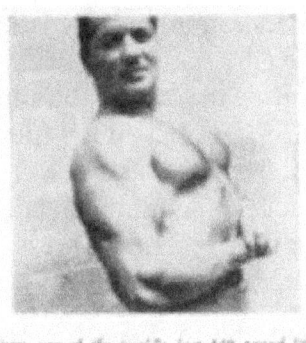

Eddie Harrison, one of the world's best 148 pound lifters, hand balancer and all around athlete, demonstrating the upright rowing motion and the two hands press.

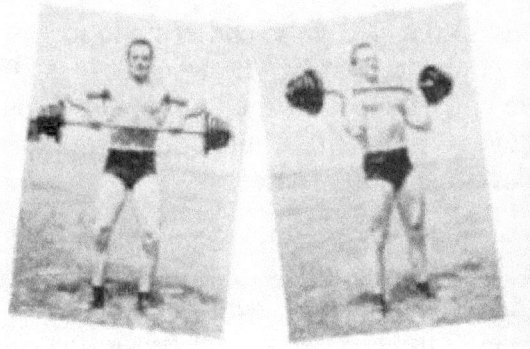

Aside from these movements a great deal of arm benefit is obtained from all forms of cleaning and snatching. But this has been covered in other chapters. The Triceps exercise while leaning and straightening the arms behind the back may easily be taken care of with a bar bell as well as with dumbells. But the principal exercise for the upper arm is pressing in its various forms. The military press is the best known of these. With the body held erect or in the military position, the weight is pressed to arm's length overhead. No movement of the body is permitted. The weight must be elevated solely with the strength of shoulders, arms and allied groups.

The continental press, which permits the body to be inclined as far as your flexibility will permit to the rear, develops the arms from about the same position as does the floor dip. But it is much more easily made progressive and is more beneficial for the remainder of the body. The floor press does not permit nearly as great a range of movement as the box or bench press, but much more weight can be handled so it has unusual advantages. The box or bench press permits a greater range of movement and the handling of much more weight in repetition pressing than does the military press so it creates a fine effect for the upper arm.

Side pressing can even more easily be practiced with a bar bell than with a dumbell. Differentiate between the side press and the more advanced bent press by holding the bell off the body in the side press and keeping the legs straight throughout. In bent pressing, the weight is rested upon the hip and the body, especially the Latissimus, throughout the various stages of the lift. Either of these exercises is a splendid developer for the Triceps.

Kindly remember that any movement in which a weight is lifted overhead has its benefit for the development of the back of the arm. The press behind neck, the jerk behind neck and holding the weight overhead provide a fair measure of development for the Triceps as do all lifting movements—the repetition two hand and one hand jerks in particular. In the snatches the back of the arm has little to do but hold the weight overhead.

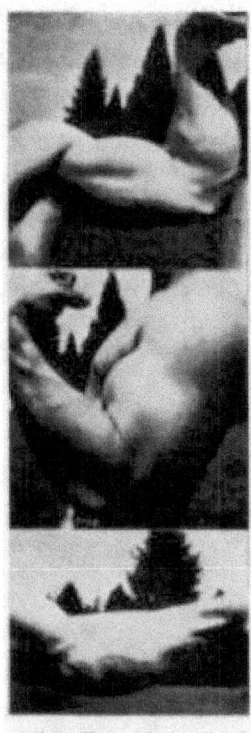

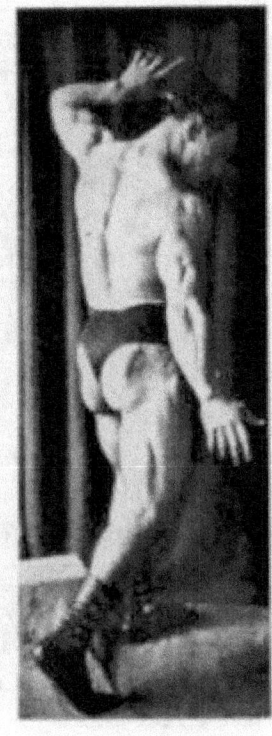

Above: The arm of Johnny Terpak.

Tony Massimo at right, so posed that he shows his great arms to good advantage.

How to Obtain Your Biggest Measurements

THE tape measure is a usual part of the body builder's equipment. It is natural that we should desire to measure; in fact that is the best means of measuring the progress or lack of progress which results from a particular form of exercise. When our measurements improve, as shown by the tape, we know that we are on the right track and can continue with the particular training procedure being followed at the moment. If weight and muscle gaining are the desire, ever bigger measurements register sure progress. And if reducing the waistline of one who is overweight is the aim, the tape measure once again is an infallible means to register progress.

It's necessary that we know how to measure so that we will all use the same methods and know how we compare in measurement and proportions with others. I have always been impressed with the very small arm measurements published for the big heavyweight fighters. The only explanation I can think of would be that the arm measurement of the straight arm was taken. In body building circles it has long been customary to measure the upper arm flexed to its limit at its biggest point to obtain the largest possible measurement. The forearm measurement is taken contracted but straight.

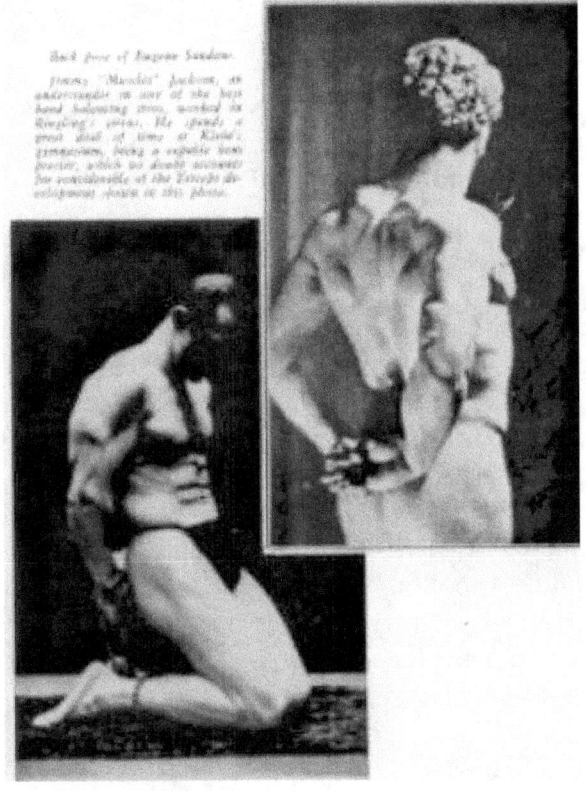

One of the largest forearms on record belonged to Appollon of France. His forearm was reported to be 17 3/4 inches straight and 19 inches flexed. If you measure your forearm straight, and another individual measures the forearm flexed, it's evident that you could not hope to compare favorably in muscular size with the other fellow. Arthur Dandurand, the French-Canadian, who was one of the best a few years ago, had one of the finest pairs of forearms ever to grace the human body. They reached what had been considered to be the ultimate in development—7 inches, or comparatively small wrist, and a remarkable 14 inch forearm development. There has been a great deal of exaggeration of measurements, especially of the arm. One "train you by mail" advertiser of the present claims a weight of 178 pounds and a forearm measurement of 14 3/4 inches. I weigh 250 at present, have had better than fair forearms for some years, as evidenced by my ten consecutive back hand curls of no pounds and a single success with 140, but my forearm has never been much past 14 inches. In fact while a group of our lifters were in Cuba this last winter my arm was measured at 14 inches cold, or as cold as one could be in such a hot climate. By cold I mean without the pumping action of the blood as a result of exercise. A photo was taken that day while I was bent pressing only the moderate weight of 205. But my arm looked a bit like some one's leg, and still measured just 14 inches. The other chap I mentioned, " the train you by mail" professor, had his picture on the wall with the forearm measurement of 14 1/2 inches. There is a limit to the size of measurements which can be obtained for a certain bodyweight. Appollon was a giant of a man, and could easily have had such tremendous measurements for he has long been famed for his hand and arm strength. But Dandurand's measurement is the best authentic measurement I have ever heard of and he weighed around two hundred pounds.

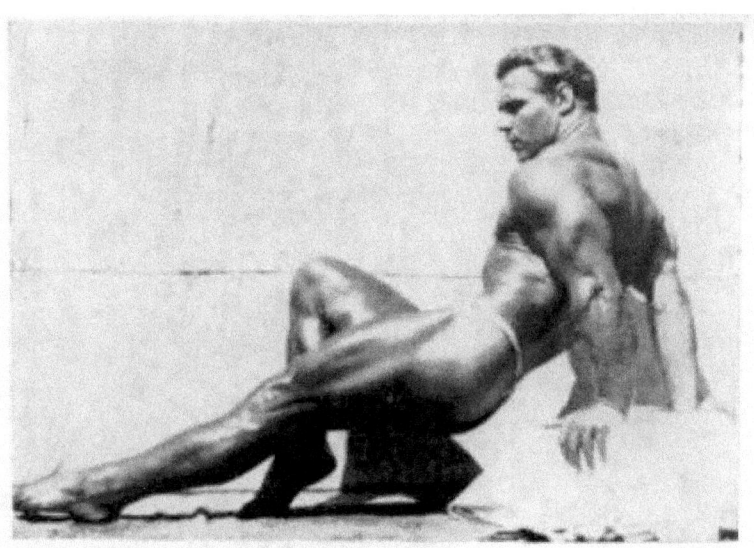

Nosseir the great Egyptian, who held the world's two hands snatch and the two hands clean and jerk record, a record that has only been bested by one pound in the many years which have passed since his establishment of that record, is credited with a wrist of 7 3/4 inches and a forearm of 14 1/2. This sounds authentic, for Nosseir won the Olympic 181 pound title in 1928, proof that he was not naturally a big-boned man. Later, through continued lifting practice, he greatly increased his bodyweight and with it an increase in measurements was inevitable. Zbyszko had a tremendous wrist of 8.6 and a forearm of 16.8.

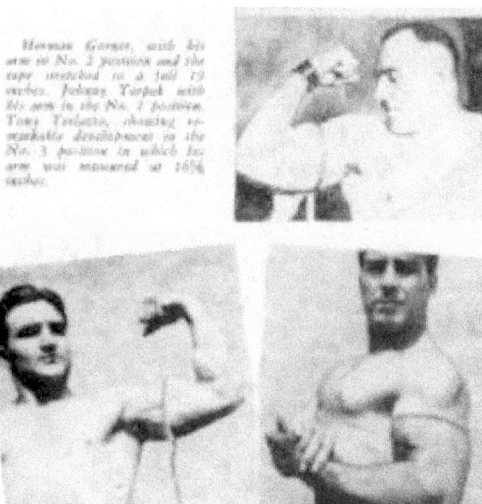

Most men believe that the size of the wrist controls the size of the measurements in the upper arm. It has been proven on numerous occasions that the size of the wrist can be greatly increased through training. The bone of course will not grow, but the muscles and tendons can be developed to a huge size which has resulted in an increase of more than an inch in wrist size of a man well past the voting age.

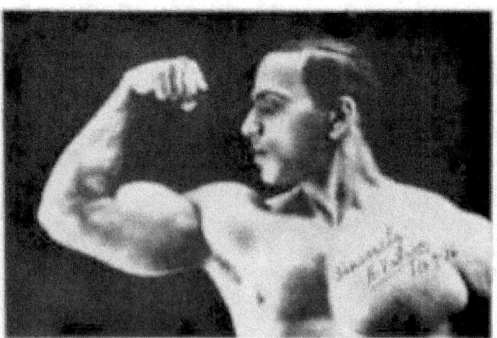

K. V. Iyer of Bangalore, Ind., a tow ball man who has a just claim to the title, "Best built man in all India."

In measuring the arms the average enthusiast who has become impressed with the idea that a big arm measure-

170

ment is a certain criterion of strength—the most important of all measurements—will resort to all sorts of maneuvers to make his arm measurement as large as possible. He will pass the tape around the arm at an angle instead of directly around the arm as it should be. There is a temptation to do this, for with many men's arms the biggest part of the Biceps is close to the Deltoid and not in line with the big swelling sweep of the Triceps muscle. Increased development will round out the Biceps and make possible the greatest possible arm measurement without the necessity of slanting the tape.

A slanted tape will show a half inch or at times a full inch more than the man is entitled to. He is just kidding himself, making believe that the arm is larger than it is. The arm measurements, like those of the leg, should always be taken at right angles to the bone.

You should get a guaranteed tape. There have been errors ranging from 1/2 inch to 2 inches in a 36 inch tape. A metal tape of good construction is more likely to be correct. If the cloth tape you employ stretches, you are cutting down the size of your measurements, and if it shrinks from constant measuring after exercise, the result of perspiration, it will make your measurements bigger than they really are. Such a tape is usually greatly wrinkled and some enthusiasts hold the tape as loosely as possible which again will not result in a fair measurement. On the other hand, a man is entitled to every ten thousandth of an inch of arm measurement he has won through his aspirations and his perspiration. Some years ago I had written in glowing terms of the splendid arm development of Wally Zagurski. It was very close to 17 inches at that time as I had measured it. One of our competitors, who was suffering under the influence of the "green-eyed monster " at the time, measured Wally's arm at only 16 inches. He measured it cold, with a steel tape, and not only did not seek the biggest part of the arm, but

171

tightened the tape so that it cut deeply into the muscle. This was not fair, and was done only to discredit Wally's published measurements. Each body building enthusiast should strive to give himself every fraction of an inch of additional arm size he can measure with the tape, but avoid any subterfuges which would not come under the classification of absolute fairness.

While not as difficult to keep the tape at the proper point when you are measuring your own arm as when measuring the thigh, or the chest, it is difficult and there are few persons who have the dexterity to handle the tape entirely unassisted. You can alleviate the difficulty in measuring the arm if you will procure a small metal ring which should be sewed into the end of the tape in such a way that the outermost end of the ring will be just even with the former edge of the tape. Pass the tape through the ring, so as to make a loop and pass it over your arm. With a tape adjusted in this manner you can obtain exact arm measurements and more definitely measure your progress. You won't experience the discouragement when a faulty measurement apparently proves that your arm has not grown, or an exaggerated measurement fills you with elation which will cause future disappointment. It will cost you more to obtain a tape such as I am describing, but it won't cost as much as a steel tape and if it is a good one it will serve as well as a steel tape.

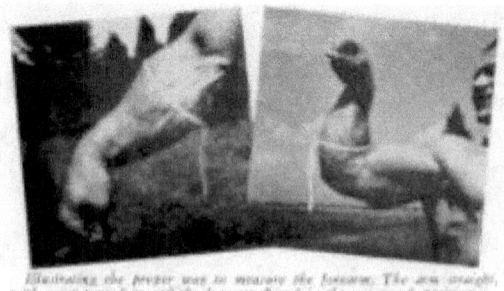

Illustrating the proper way to measure the forearm. The arm straight, with wrist turned in and the forearm flexed in the measured position.

In preparing to take the measurement of the upper arm, it is your privilege to measure when the arm has been warmed or pumped up with blood as the result of vigorous arm exercise. This will add from a quarter inch to a half inch to the normal measurement. The arm is usually larger in the morning, and concentrated curling exercises at that time will result in the largest possible measurement. Your ability at controlling the Biceps will have much to do with the magnitude of the measurement you are able to obtain. Before measuring the arm you should go through the motions of straightening and flexing the arm until it feels fatigued. This will draw blood to the Biceps but it will also permit you to display a much more prominent bump. There are several ways of measuring the arm: Cold, and after exercise, and in a number of positions. To simplify arm measurement in the future, I suggest, when arm measurements are taken and reported to me or to others, that the notation " taken cold " or taken after exercise be offered, and whether it was taken in positions i, 2, or 3. No. 1 Position, with the upper arm held out from the shoulder, elbow level with the shoulder, forearm at right angles to the upper arm. Position No. 2, with the upper arm in the same position, but with the forearm drawn back until the clenched fist almost touches the shoulder. No. 3: The arm at side, against the body, upper arm in a perpendicular position, forearm at right angles to it.

There is another position, in which it is possible to obtain the largest measurement with some men's arms, which we are disregarding because it is not a natural position and there is considerable difficulty obtaining a fair measurement in such a position. That is, with the elbow held high, almost directly above the body, the elbow against the side of the head, and the hand drawn so far back that it rests upon the nape of the neck.

I find in checking articles in magazines and chapters in books of years ago, which deal with arm development and measurements, that nearly every writer explained to his readers that the arm was biggest when held in our No. 1 Position. It was explained that the arm was largest when the forearm was at right angles to the upper arm, because the Triceps, being nearly twice as large as the Biceps, is almost completely relaxed when the hand is brought to the shoulder. It was admitted that this position with the hand close to the shoulder was the best position for Biceps display, but as the Biceps was the smaller of the two muscle groups, more was lost in Triceps size than was gained in Biceps display in the No. 2 Position. Therefore, in their opinions, the largest measurement would be obtained with the forearm at right angles to the upper arm.

I do not know whether these men were theorists only, whether they did not measure other arms, or found their own arm to be ?o constructed that the largest measurements were obtained in the No. 1 Position, or if they just read what some other man had written and expressed the same belief in their own books and articles. I don't believe that arms have changed in shape materially in the last twenty-five to fifty years.

In another chapter I have discussed the largest arms, but, to illustrate, will supply heavyweight champion Steve Stanko's arm measurements in the various positions. To check the theory of the old time writers I had all the members of the York Bar Bell Weight Lifting Team measure their arms with John Grimek, Johnny Terpak and Tony Terlazzo taking the measurements. And we found, without exception, that each man's arm was largest in the No. 3 Position, next largest in No. 2 and smallest in No. 1. There was as much as one inch difference between No. 1 and No. 2. To be really sure I measured a number of arms of men who were rather meagerly developed, and found that the rule held good in their cases too, as I will explain at greater length in another chapter.

Steve's upper arm straight measured 16 1/2 inches. In Position No. 1 we found it to be 17 1/4 inches, in Position No. 2, 18 inches, and in Position No. 3, 18 1/2 inches. His forearm straight was 14 3/4 and in the gooseneck, flexed position, 15 3/4.

It has long been customary to take the forearm measurement with the arm extended, although it may be hardened and the clenched fist turned in. The measurement should be found to be largest at a point about two inches below the elbow joint. If a man is very thin he can expect to have his largest measurement right at the elbow, but if he is well developed the forearm forms a big curve so that the thickest part of the arm will be well below the elbow. The really well-developed forearm will swell out like a leg of lamb or of beef.

The big professional measurements you normally read about are taken with the forearm flexed, the upper arm straight out from the body and the forearm held with the wrist in the gooseneck position. Joe Nordquest, great old time strong man, who established a floor press record of 388 pounds and a bent press record of 277%, had a forearm which, when measured straight, stretched the tape at 14V2 inches and at 16^3A inches when flexed.

While measurements are always interesting, the development of the arm, the relation of the forearm and upper arm muscles as compared to the wrist and elbow, will

make possible a splendid muscular display which does not require a tape to prove the excellence of the development. The small-boned man with moderate arm measurements will have a finer appearing arm than will the man with big bones and a huge wrist, who can display greater measurements but does not have the shapeliness and the apparent

175

size. Most of us are controlled to a certain extent by heredity, by the bone size we inherit. But unlike the bulldog which is always massively developed if it does nothing but spend its life chained to a kennel, and the greyhound which remains a great hound in development even though it spends its life as a sled dog, people are of such mixed ancestry that they can obtain an outstanding development in every case by training hard and intelligently, and following the rules of health.

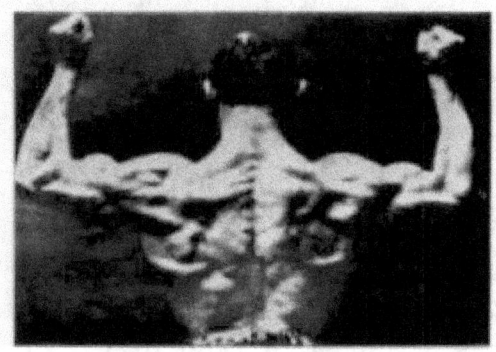

Anatomy and Development of The Forearm

A BIG upper arm is the pride and joy of many a strength athlete's life, while he is prone to forget the wrist and the forearm. Yet they are just as important in providing an attractive development as is the better known Biceps. The Superinator muscles, in particular, of the upper forearm are fastened well up the Humerus bone, and apparently shorten as well as thicken the upper arm to add to its development.

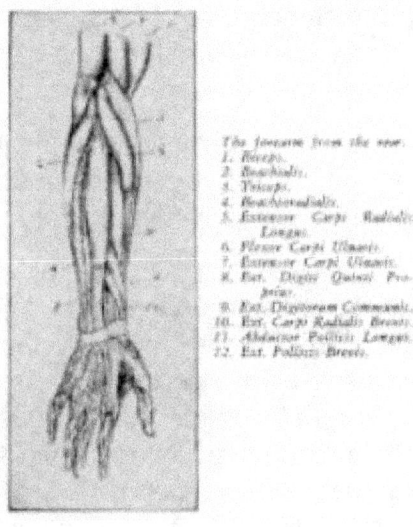

The forearm from the rear.
1. Biceps.
2. Brachialis.
3. Triceps.
4. Brachioradialis.
5. Extensor Carpi Radialis Longus.
6. Flexor Carpi Ulnaris.
7. Extensor Carpi Ulnaris.
8. Ext. Digiti Quinti Proprius.
9. Ext. Digitorum Communis.
10. Ext. Carpi Radialis Brevis.
11. Abductor Pollicis Longus.
12. Ext. Pollicis Brevis.

Every time we pick up any sort of an object it calls for not only the strength of the grip but results in forearm development. Many salesmen have a grip and forearm development far out of proportion to the development of the rest of the body because they habitually carry their sample case, changing from hand to hand, and also clasp hands with a great many prospects, exerting considerable force in an endeavor to create a favorable impression. A grip alone cannot be developed; it comes as a result of forearm strength, and of course forearm strength and development result from picking up, carrying objects, lifting and bending of the forearms.

We could delve very deeply into the anatomy of the forearm, but I do not believe it is necessary in a book such as this. The student who wishes more can so easily obtain it from any well-known text book of anatomy. The muscles of the forearm are classified as Pronators, Flexors and Extensors. The Flexors bend the forearm upon the upper arm, the Extensors straighten the arm, while the Pronators are the muscles of rotation, those which turn or twist the arms. In examining the front of the forearm, we find four separate muscles having a common place of origin on the Humerus bone, near the elbow joint. They form the bulk of the well-developed forearm as they divide and spread.

The canoe like muscle which gives the greatest bulk and roundness to the forearm when straight, and is even more forcibly evident when flexed, is the second from the inside of the four muscles.

The muscles on the outside of the forearm are seven in number and included among them is the Superinator Longus, which in my own case made itself so evident at one time through a light strain from back hand curling. There is the Brachioradialis, which is the most important of the Extensor muscles of the forearm. Beside it is another Extensor muscle designed to cooperate with the Superinator called Extensor Carpi Radialis Longus. One of the most unusual features of the forearms are their ability to twist, to exert great force while turning. The Superinator Longus muscle and its closest associate have a great spiral twist in their formation. This muscle has its inception at the Humerus bone, at a point just underneath the Biceps muscle. From that point of origin it extends or twists over the outside of the elbow joint where it becomes fastened to the front of the forearm. Without doubt, this Superinator Longus muscle is the most important muscle of the forearm. It performs more functions than any other forearm muscle, or perhaps any other one muscle of the body. It serves equally well at rotation, flexion and very powerfully extends or straightens the arm. Being so powerful, and serving such a variety of purposes, it naturally presents a fine appearance in the well-developed arm. It adds greatly to the breadth of the arm, especially when viewed from the side.

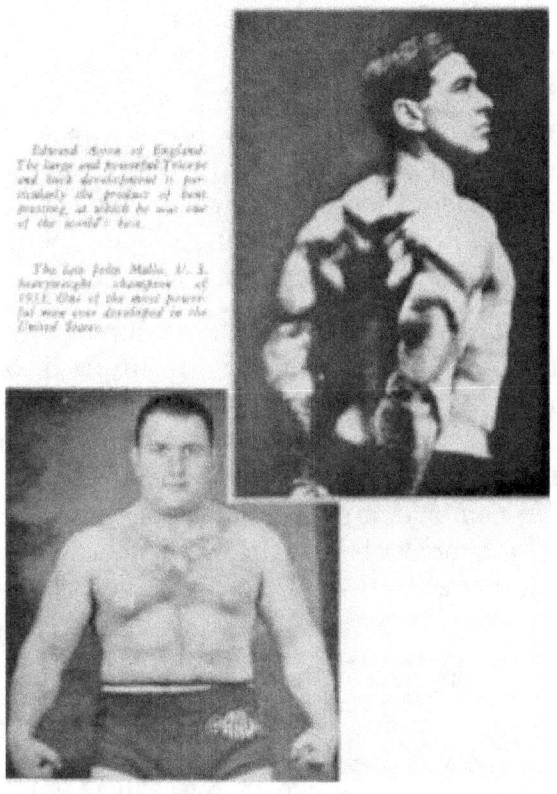

Edward Aston of England. The large and powerful Triceps and back development is particularly the product of bent pressing, at which he was one of the world's best.

The late John Mollo, U. S. heavyweight champion of 1933. One of the most powerful men ever developed in the United States.

This is the muscle which is most evident in the development of laborers, mechanics, farmers and others who frequently carry heavy objects. When I was about fourteen years of age, and ambitious to develop muscle, but having little to show for my pains, I would note the unusual development of the Superinator Longus on the arm of an older schoolmate who lived on a nearby farm. I did not know the name of the muscle but I saw its fine development and noticed that muscle on the arms of other hard-working men many times after that. You can find this muscle on your own arm by first curling the hand until it rests on the chest. Contract it still farther by pushing with the free hand and you will see and feel it very noticeably displayed at the side of the elbow.

Keeping the arm in the same position, twist the wrist and feel the action of this muscle; note how firmly it becomes tensed. And when a weight is lifted overhead, and held at arm's length, it is this muscle which performs a great deal of the work of straightening the arm and holding the heavy weight overhead. Then it cooperates with the Triceps muscle, just as in back hand curling it helps the Brachialis Anticus, and in front curling, assists the Biceps.

The other muscles of the forearm are principally Flexors and Superinators and their only aid in lifting or holding a weight overhead is to serve as balancers. The muscles of the front of the arm are Flexors and are brought into play most fully with movements which bend the arm at the elbow. The contraction of these Flexors is even more evident when any object is raised toward the shoulder, while holding the wrist downward, so that it forms a goose or swan neck.

Beginners in physical training, who have not received development from hard work, are always most deficient in Flexor and Superinator development. With the body builder who only performs one or two exercises there will be a lack of development in these muscles also. The size of the forearm will increase with the years, for while the young man may have well shaped forearms, they seldom are large in size. But with the passing of years and increased use, they will gain a certain adiposity of tissue which will account for much larger size.

It has seemed to me that thinner arms, with very prominent veins showing, always attracted more favorable attention than bigger arms without the veins clearly defined. Vascularity this is called, and the uninitiated will believe that they are corded muscles in the arms of the man who possesses them. This vascularity accounts for a great deal of the development of some men's arms. They usually greatly amplify the size of the inside of the forearm, provide bulk on the outside of the forearm just above the wrist and farther up the arm where the Brachioradialis bulges out. It's quite evident that the old timers felt that vascularity of the veins was an important part of development, for in some of the old pictures the veins were touched up to add to their impressive appearance. There are some who believe that the appearance of these veins is unsightly, but there are just as many who admire them. The men who have prominent veins are usually those who at times work continuously with their arms, carrying heavy objects for considerable distances. The forearm muscles are tensed, the blood must go on its merry way, and the veins become enlarged so that they can pass on the outside of the tensed muscle. Before posing the forearms for a picture, the veins will become especially prominent when a few warming up exercises are practiced.

Tendons, ligaments and other muscular attachments have a tendency to become thicker and more prominent as a man advances in years. This, with the addition of more prominent blood vessels and thickening of their walls, causes the mature man of strength to frequently have more impressive forearms than the younger man.

All body culturists should remember that there is more to the arm than just muscle. Ligaments, tendons, other attachments, fascia, nerves, bones, blood vessels, skin, and a certain amount of fatty tissue make up the weight and development of the body.

The best forearms are the result of working them in conjunction with the upper arms. So don't expect too much in the way of development by practicing exercises designed to benefit the forearm alone. As I have sought to prove, the best arms are the result of all around training, the handling of heavy weights, and of course the forearms, grip and wrist are the result of such training procedure also. If you will practice the regular course and then, as a means of specialization, practice some of the exercises which involve more particularly the forearms, such as the back hand curl and the twisting movements, which are not experienced in any of the regular lifting movements, you will develop all the muscles of the forearms.

The handling of thick bars will bring the forearm muscles into play in an entirely different manner—some men having much more ability to handle big weights with thick bars than small ones. I find that I can bent press a great deal better with my stage bell, which has a three inch handle, than with the Olympic standard bells which are i Vio inches in diameter. It gives one more to press against and my best record is 23V2 pounds higher with the big bell than with the Olympic standard—240 as compared to 263 3/4.

The forearms can stand a great deal of hard work when once they are accustomed to it. It is necessary for you to give them plenty of work if you hope to reach nearly the ultimate in strength and development. So many exercises have been offered in this book that more explanation of the development of the forearm would be in the nature of repetition.

Developing A Powerful Grip

DID you ever shake hands with a man whose hand felt like he had just placed a cold piece of meat in your hand—cold, clammy, no life? It was White who wrote of former President Wilson: "When you meet the man he will lay his hand in yours and you will think at once of a dead, cold mackerel." Woodrow Wilson was a fine man. He had many friends, but was heartily disliked by those who knew him but slightly. He had too much handicap to overcome as a result of the bad impression his cold manner and lifeless hand grip created at first. It's important that all of us, especially those whose living depends upon creating a good first impression, such as salesmen, put our best foot forward at all times. If you have a fine, warm, strong handclasp, there is little doubt that it will create a very favorable impression always and have an important bearing on the happiness and success you obtain from life. There is no doubt that the nature of one's handclasp bears such great importance that it has been known to make and break men. Frequently you read in literature, "His handclasp was firm, warm and friendly; one knew him instantly as a man who could be depended upon." Or "He was untrustworthy, had a loose, cold, clammy handclasp and could not look you straight in the eye." And so on and so on.

On the other hand, there is just as great a nuisance in meeting the person who grasps your hand, grits his teeth, rises on his toes and bears down with every ounce of strength at his command in the effort to grind the bones in your hand to powder. He has a good grip and knows it, seizes every opportunity to demonstrate it, until all and sundry detest the sight of him.

You may have tried some of the exercises which I will now offer, although some of them will be entirely new to you. In any event if you include some of these exercises in your regular training program for six to twelve weeks you are sure to improve your forearms and have a well developed pair of phenomenally strong hands.

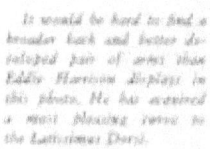

It would be hard to find a broader back and better developed pair of arms than Eddie Harrison displays in this photo. He has acquired a most pleasing curve to the Latissimus Dorsi.

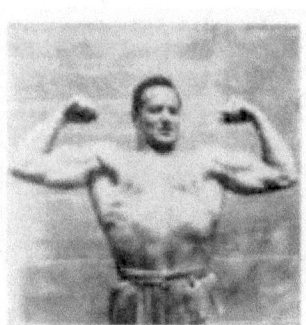

It is possible to classify the various exercises for the hands and I believe it would be beneficial for you to include each in its own category. I shall therefore list them as the Bending and Breaking Group, the Tearing Group, the Pinching Group and the Gripping Group. While there is a marked difference among the above allocations, there is of course some overlapping. However, it will demonstrate its value as I describe the different exercises; moreover, it will provide a means whereby the exercise enthusiast may select a different group for each exercise period of the week and thus reach the muscles in diversified manner.

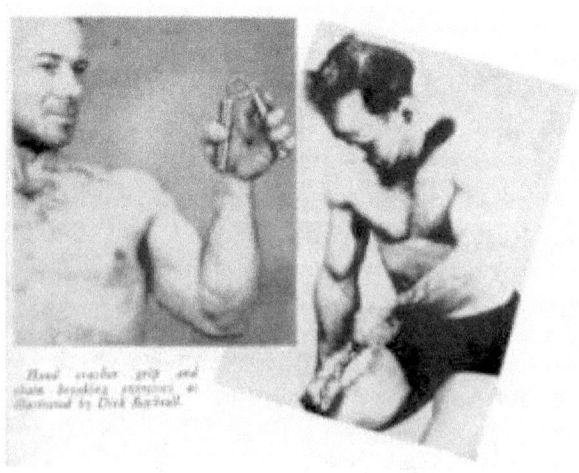

Hand crusher grip and chain breaking exercises as illustrated by Dick Bachtell.

184

In the first division, the Bending and Breaking Group, one will immediately realize the necessity of strong, tough hands, both of which can be secured in a few weeks' time. Probably more than in any other of the groups, the shoulders, chest and back muscles will come in for a share of the exercises which develop the grip. The very nature of the exercises of this section causes the muscles of the upper body to pull and push and twist in most any direction. One thing you should remember at all times: The BEST exercises are those which bring into play the largest group of muscles at one time.

You should procure some strap iron and some jack chains. They'll not only help you become strong but through their use you'll develop a reputation as a really strong man. You'll be asked to give demonstrations at banquets, social gatherings and business meetings. You will surprise your friends and business associates who don't know that you have been taking "iron pills" for some time. You should obtain a piece of strap iron six to eight feet in length. Depending upon your present strength, you can start with iron varying in width from 1 to 2 1/2 inches and the thickness that experimentation shows you capable of handling. While you are at the hardware store selecting the strap iron, also obtain some spikes of various kinds (you will quickly learn to bend them too) and some jack chains. This is made in several sizes. You can start with the smallest. The second size is the sort of material used with the York Head Strap. There are at least three larger sizes that you can learn to break. After you have bent the strap iron, you need not discard it, for you will obtain additional exercise by straightening it to use again. The procedure of exercising with the strap iron is simplicity itself. First bend one end at right angles; four to six inches will be sufficient. It's better to make this initial bend in a vise. Then place one foot on the bend in order to hold it firmly to the floor, and placing the left forearm against the iron, start bending the top half of the bar over it by pushing hard with the right hand. With a little practice you can learn to make some fancy scroll work in just a few minutes' time. Don't forget to practice bending the iron over both arms to assure yourself of equal development. As a strength demonstration, heavier bars may be bent by placing them on your head or in your mouth, having assistants hang on the ends of them to pull them down. Of course you should wrap a handkerchief around the bar to protect your teeth, otherwise you may be faced with a large dental bill.

In bending spikes it's usually customary to bend them slightly over the leg just above the knee, then apply your strength as is done with the Giant Crusher Grip, bending them until the ends nearly touch. With a light enough spike you can learn to make the entire bend with your hands. It requires practice, during which a certain amount of knack is developed, and of course strength. Bending spikes is always quite impressive. There is another feat which is startling to the spectators and splendid from the development standpoint—driving spikes through a board. Start first with a soft, one inch straight grained board; sharpen the spike with a file, wrap a handkerchief carefully around the head end of the spike, extend the other between the second and third fingers; the head of the spike is of course held against the palm of the hand; clench the fist, and then strike a hard pushing blow to begin. In a comparatively short time you will acquire the ability to drive a spike repeatedly through a two inch plank. It does not require a great deal of bodily strength to perform these feats. Anyone can learn to do them with practice.

One of the best ways to break a chain is to fasten it to a ring in a heavy board. Stand on the board, then loop the chain around the dumbell or bar bell bar. The chain should be just large enough that the bar is slightly above the knees. Before preparing to lift, twist the chain once; this should place one link in a position to break before the rest. Chain breaking is difficult if this twist is not present; otherwise five or six links may stretch at one time, making it difficult to have enough range in movement with chest expansion to break the chain, and while lifting with the back and arms, the body may find itself in a position where the full strength of back and legs can not be applied.

I can break the first three sizes of jack chain without a twist on my chest, but need this on the largest linked chains. I have a pretty good range of expansion and contraction of the Latissimus muscles in particular. But the man without so large a chest, or so much expansion, must concentrate all his effort upon a single link as is done in twisting the chain.

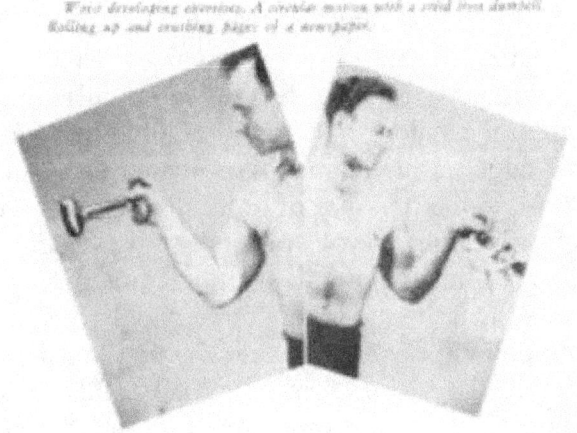

Wrist developing exercises. A circular motion with a solid iron dumbell. Rolling up and crushing pages of a newspaper.

You can make your start as a strap iron, iron bar and spike bender by training with the Giant Crusher Grip—the grip and wrist developer which is a part of the York weight training outfit well known as the Big Ten—or an Iron Shoe. These devices have a direct effect upon the muscles which are developed and required in the bending of iron bars.

A rather impressive way of demonstrating your strength is the tearing of playing cards in halves, quarters and eighths, the latter being the most difficult, I assure you, even for the strongest handed person. I have heard of tearing cards into eighths, but it has never been my pleasure to see it legitimately demonstrated. I say legitimately, because there are various types of playing cards, the very cheapest kind being quite easy for a strong handed man to tear. Moreover, it is the practice of some so-called strong men to bake the cards in an oven, thus thoroughly drying out the cardboard which destroys its fibre sufficiently to almost cause the cards to fall apart. Large catalogues and phone books prove accessible material for the practice of tearing. The companies who put out these books no doubt would appreciate it a great deal if you use last year's books.

With each successive pack of cards or phone books you tear, you will learn new tricks which will add to the smoothness of performing the tearing operation. There are certain details to be observed, which, when put into practice, will aid you in the demonstration of tearing. With either cards or catalogues it is absolutely necessary that a good stiff edge be maintained. And when once the tear is started, turn on the pressure in order that the tear will carry completely through. If you are not strong enough to tear them apart while in normal position, you can slip them somewhat so that the full tear is underway before you come to the complete deck. The manner of gripping the cards is rather simple, a reversed grip being used. Place the hands over each end of the deck in a reversed position, grip the cards firmly with the fingers and the thumb, and being sure that you have a stiff edge on the cards, twist them apart. It requires strong hands to tear one deck of cards, but there are men who have torn two or three decks at one time.

I don't believe I will suggest that you try the bending and breaking of coins for the reason that so far as the U. S. coins are concerned, it is not possible to bend them apart with the hands alone. Even if it were possible, our dear old Uncle Sammy would strenuously discourage the practice.

Seriously now, I believe it would provide a pretty big order to accomplish with a quarter or a half dollar. It might be possible with a thin dime. Try fastening a half dollar in a vise and using only the thumb or the heel of the hand as a means of breaking the coin; you will see how difficult it is.

The pinching powers are most easily developed by carrying the largest plates of your bar bell by pinching them between thumb and fingers. Practice dropping them by releasing your grip and catching them again. Don't miss, for the people downstairs might complain. You will find that it will take but little of this kind of exercise to tire your arms and forearms and that of course means that good results will be obtained from the exercise. This movement will be fatiguing, especially if you are advanced to the point of using heavy plates. When you are capable of handling smooth, fifty pound plates in this style, you can be assured that you have an unusual grip. At a lifting show that I attended a few years ago, one of the loaders who was justly proud of his grip, while preparing to weigh a bar bell that had been lifted, was forced to dismantle the weights on account of the low position of the scale. He picked up the two fifties, one with the pinch grip of each hand, and walking past George Zottman, the man who is credited with originating the twisting curl, said, " George, how do you like this stunt? Could you do that?" George didn't say a word: Standing as he was with his coat on, serving as one of the officials, he walked over to the plates, picked them up as the loader had done, but he muscled them out. This was a feat and the loader and we who saw him perform this feat were rendered speechless.

Dave Stone, the Maine strong boy, was one of the first to succeed in two hands snatching a pair of fifty pound plates using only the pinch grip. This great feat has been duplicated on several occasions since—proof that strong-handed men are still being developed in this country. And when you reach the point of being able to carry a pair of seventy-five pound plates with the pinch grip, then you can feel that you are near the top of the iron man profession.

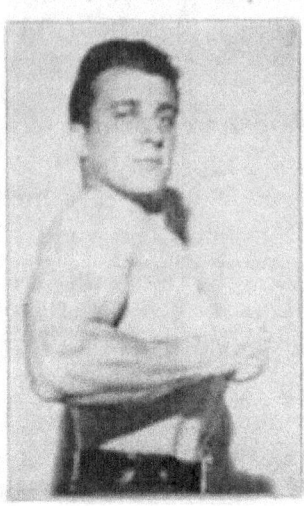

Jack Mitchell, of Raleigh, North Carolina, a weight trained man who has one of the best arms.

Warren Lincoln Travis, who spent so many years at Coney Island performing very heavy supporting and lifting feats, back, harness, and hip lifts, had a few feats which stopped everyone who tried them. He had weights so arranged that they just suited him, which made it difficult for the other fellow with larger or smaller hands to exactly duplicate. But they were great feats just the same. He would lift a large block weight with just the first knuckle of his thumb and finger. He would lift a ring to which a weight was suspended by the extended forefinger, knuckles up. John Davis was the only man who duplicated this particular feat at Coney Island. Travis did a lot of finger lifting too. One night at nearby Harrisburg I saw him perform a two finger lift with 830 pounds. But this sort of a feat isn't much fun. The padded ring which supported the weight cut his fingers to the bone.

If you desire, you can easily make yourself a pinch grip developer. Secure a piece of 2 by 4 about 18 inches long.

Drill two holes in it through which you can pass two strong cords to suspend a dumbell which you can load to the proper weight for the gripping exercise. Another means of developing the pinching powers, and one little used, is the practice of bending pop bottle caps between the thumb and index finger. It may be necessary for you to practice other exercises before you are strong enough to accomplish this one, but it will prove a valuable means of further strengthening the muscles we are considering in this chapter.

Most of the exercises I have offered can be used in strong man exhibitions. They have great development value in addition to building a reputation as a strength performer. They will help you develop a super grip, such as few men possess.

Dead lifting in both the regular and reversed grip styles is a sure way of securing Herculean gripping powers, especially when very heavy weights are employed. In exercises such as the deep knee bend, the half bend, the rise on toes, if you are really ambitious to build a strong grip, you can hold the weight with your hands. Recently I offered a series of compound exercises, which, while designed to develop all the muscles, will give the grip and forearms plenty of work. The first night I tried this movement with 125 pounds—ten two hand curls, ten two hand presses, ten deep knee bends, ten rowing motions and ten dead lifts. I got through the first series with just a little faster breathing. Then I reduced the weight to a hundred pounds and performed ten back hand curls, ten press behind neck, ten deep knee bends on toes, ten upright rowing motions and ten stiff legged dead lifts. Half way through the second course I was breathing like I had just finished a mile run, and my forearms ached almost like a toothache. So it's sure that such a stiff program will bring real results.

In any exercise program, the regular dead lift, the Jefferson lift, front and back hand curl, the Zottman curl, rowing motion and repetition snatches will provide a wonderful workout for your hands, wrists and forearms. You can invest in a few various sized pipes to thrust over your bar bell between the collars, and this will further strengthen your wrists. Almost without exception you will notice that leading lifters have strong hands and powerful muscular forearms which look big from every angle. This is the direct result of having handled heavy weights in their training. Those among them who practice dead hang snatches and cleans have remarkably developed forearms and hands.

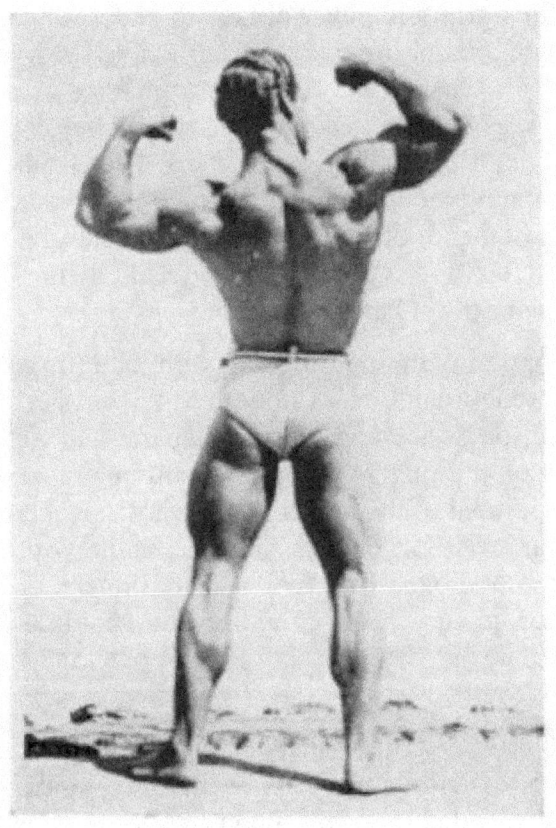

The magnificent back of John Grimek.

My father had the most powerful grip and hand development I have ever seen. I think that is a pretty big statement, because I know many hundreds of strong men personally. But I have never seen anything that remotely approached his hand and wrist development. When his fist was clenched it reminded one more of a sixteen pound shot than anything human. Squeeze your hand by clenching your fist; turn it forward slightly. What sort of development do you see on the wrist? In spite of years of rowing, pulling on oars and lifting, I have no great development there. But my father had a hump of muscle and a deep hole which must have been an inch and a half apart. He was justly proud of his grip and never ceased to endeavor to improve it. He made a habit of walking from where we lived, about three miles to his office. He made a practice of squeezing something as he walked—a pair of rubber balls, a tin tobacco box, a big ball of newspapers. Every time his foot on the gripping side touched the ground he would squeeze and as the other foot touched he would relax his grip. He kept this up for years and it resulted in the most extraordinary grip I have ever seen.

Floor dipping with the fingers, with one finger or one thumb on each hand, as is done by the best performers— men like Bob Jones and Val de Genaro,—or actual hand balancing on the fingers is sure to result in a most outstanding development of the hands and forearms. Rope climbing, tug of war, walking on the hands, chinning from various sized horizontal bars, with two or more fingers, or even one if you become very good, chinning while holding to a joist, two by four, or two by six, takes power and provides resulting benefit.

The hand crusher grip, which is a part of each Home Gym, and can be had separately, is a fine developer. Winding weights suspended by a cord upon a roller, such as is a part of the Big Ten Special, is one of the best grip and hand developers known. Moderate practice of the exercises I have suggested will eventually lead to truly impressive forearms, strong hands and wrists with power to spare.

One Hundred and One Dumbell Exercises

1. Regular two arm curl.

2. Alternate curl—palms up.

3. Back hand curl.

4. Back hand curl, alternate.

5. Curl with thumbs up.

6. Right hand curl.

7. Left hand curl.

8. Front curl, leaning.

9. Back curl, leaning.

10. Alternate curl and press.

11. Upright rowing motion.

12. Leaning over rowing motion.

13. Alternate rowing motion, leaning.

14. Arms swing to side while leaning.

15. Arms held to front while leaning and rotating.

16. Swinging from overhead far to the left, down and up to the right. Then reverse.

17. Swinging from position at side of foot to overhead, down to side of other foot and continue.

18. Zottman or twisting curl.

19. Triceps exercise while straightening arms to back of body while leaning forward.

20. Press while squatting on toes.

21. Press while rising from squat.

22. Lateral raise.

23.　　Forward raise.

24.　　Alternate forward raise.

25.　　Wrestler's bridge and press two dumbells.

26.　　Flying exercise with dumbells while lying upon bench, back down. Keeping arms bent at elbows, draw the bells together over body until they touch, extend as far to side as possible while keeping elbows bent. Then back to center, keep flying or flapping the arms like wings, varying the position of the hands from near the face to well down the thighs.

27.　　Lateral raise while lying.

28.　　Pull over lying.

29.　　Revolving dumbells while lying. Starting with the bells on the thighs, knuckles up, start to bring the arms toward the face, keeping them close to body, crossing arms as face is reached and going back to the original position with a wide sweep of the arms away from the body.

30.　　Lying on back hold both arms straight overhead. Turn both hands far to the left, then back to center, then far to the right.

31.　　Lying on back, spread arms far to side in line with shoulders, cross them over chest and then back to position with arms extended.

32.　　Alternate curl and press to arm's length back of head while lying.

33.　　Two hands military press dumbells.

34.　　One hand military press, left.

35.　　Military press with opposite arm.

36.　　Side press, right.

37.　　Side press, left.

38.   Two hands press while lying.

39.   Alternate press while lying.

40.   Left hand swing.

41.   Right hand swing.

42.   Two hands swing.

43.   Punching movements, straight right and left.

44.   Punching movements, alternate upper cuts.

45.   Punching movements, right and left hand swing.

46.   Punching movements, right and left hook.

47.   Forward press from shoulders and twist.

48.   Hold arms out at sides, shoulder height, palms up. Curl them to position against head.

49.   Hold arms at sides, shoulder height, palms down. Curl to position beside head.

50.   Curl at shoulder height, to front, palms up.

51.   Curl at shoulder height, to front, knuckles up.

52.   Circular motion while standing. Start with bells across thighs, knuckles up. Raise the arms, keeping close to the body and knuckles front. Extend to arm's length overhead and lower with arms held out from side—similar to the position while lying on a bench but it brings different muscles into play. It's a favorite exercise of John Grimek.

53.   Alternate upright rowing motion.

54.   Hold bells at shoulder height extended to the front. Keeping them at shoulder height, extend out to side.

55.   A variation of the former exercise. Start by raising bells to the side at shoulder height, keeping arms straight. Draw them in to a position with bells touching at shoulder height in front of the body; raise to arm's length overhead,

lower to side, back to center and down. It's a very good arm and Deltoid exercise.

56. Curl up under armpits.

57. Alternate curl up under armpits.

58. Left hand bent press.

59. Right hand bent press.

60. One arm press from position at front of hip.

61. One hand side press, body held erect throughout from position at side of hip.

62. One hand side press from position with elbow at back of hip.

63. Left hand snatch.

64. Right hand snatch.

65. Left hand clean.

66. Right hand clean.

67. Left hand jerk.

68. Right hand jerk.

69. Two hands clean with dumbells.

70. Two hands jerk with dumbells.

71. Two hands continental press or push.

72. Hold bell overhead, touch toes.

73. Straddle hop with dumbells held in hands.

74. Carrying weights while running or climbing stairs.

75. Two hands snatch with dumbells.

76. Dropping and catching bell from hand to hand.

77. Two hands curl while sitting on chair.

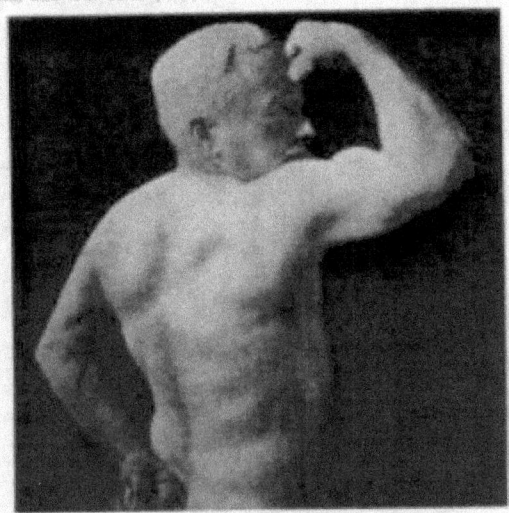

78.   Two hands press while sitting on chair.

79.   Holding elbow against side, grasping bell with right hand, twist as far as you can; grasp bar with left hand while right wrist is turned well back. Then twist bell again. Continue this movement as rapidly as possible.

80.   Holding a bell in each hand, elbows at side of body, twist back and forth until tired.

81.   Twist bell sharply around and up, releasing it and catching it. See how fast you can spin it.

82.   Sit on the floor with dumbell beside you. Holding it at arm's length raise it over the leg and set it on the floor between your legs. Then raise it again, placing it past the opposite leg. Then raise and back to center, raise and back to the outside of the leg on the lifting side. To perform this movement right you must not touch the leg or swing the weight with the body in any way.

83.   While sitting upon the floor, pull a single bell to the shoulder. Press it to arm's length three times, changing to

the right hand and press three times, keeping the bell above the head throughout the movement; continue until tired.

84.   Stand with a single bell across the front of the thigh, knuckles front. Holding the elbow stationary, curl it to the shoulder, bending the wrist well down throughout the movement so that it is in the gooseneck position. Without moving the elbow or forearm, raise and lower the bell by wrist action alone.

85.   In the same position, describe a circular motion with the power of the wrist.

86.   Sit on a chair with the dumbell, ring weight, block weight or other weight upon the floor beside you. Lift it up to table. Wait two seconds, lift it down again. Continue until tired.

87.   Another exercise which will build endurance and arm strength, too, is to perform a similar exercise while standing. Lift the dumbell from the floor to the table. Let it rest on the table for a moment, but do not let go with the hand; put

it back on the floor, lift with the other hand. Continue this movement with moderate slowness until tired.

88.   Holding the left arm at shoulder height and straight, curl the right into the shoulder, then extend the right, curling the left to the shoulder. Continue until you feel the movement.

89.   Hold a pair of moderate dumbells at arm's length, shoulder height from the sides, twist the bells back and forth until you feel the movement.

90.   Grasp the dumbell by one of the weights. Extend it out at shoulder height. With a rotary motion of the hands and wrist turn the bells round and round until you feel the movement.

91.   Hold the weights at arm's length overhead, palms facing. Lower them to shoulder height. Hold two seconds, raise back overhead and repeat. This is the well-known Crucifix lift.

92.   Hold the bells at shoulder height. Push them to arm's length, shoulder height at side, and twist. Back to the original position and repeat.

93.   Stand with the knees slightly bent. Bend down to touch the ankle with one bell, curl the other back under the armpit, back to the position of attention. Then touch the opposite hand to the opposite ankle, curling the other hand up into armpit.

94.   Hold one arm in front of body, swing to the opposite side from the shoulder, which supports the weight. Have the other arm in back and opposite its shoulder, too. Reverse the position and continue until you feel the movement.

95.   Hold the bells at shoulders, elbows front, knuckles up. Press them to arm's length overhead, keeping the knuckles up. Lower to shoulders and continue the movement.

96.   A somewhat similar movement with the elbows held out to the side. Press with knuckles up.

97.   Hold the bells at chest and lean far back, then forward until you touch toes with dumbells; back to first position and continue the movement.

98.   Sit upon the floor and go through rowing motions with

dumbells in hand. Reach far out and touch toes, bring them to chest, leaning well back, then to toes and continue the movement.

99.   Lying on your side, move the dumbell to the back, to the front and then back.

100.   Bending your knees, going into a full squat, raise the bells to shoulder height. When you come erect curl them under armpits and continue the movement.

101.   Take a pair of dumbells in your hands a bit heavier than those used in the Lateral Raise. Stand about two feet from the wall. Keeping your back flat, support yourself with back of head touching wall. Permit the bells to drop down and back until they touch behind your back. Raise from this position until they touch overhead. Lower until the bells touch behind back. This operates the arms over a much greater range and creates a favorable muscle building effect.

And here you have 101 good dumbell exercises. More than 101 if you count the opposite arm in every movement. Such a program, I am sure, is by far the most complete list of dumbell exercises ever offered. You have enough here to provide endless variety, to develop the muscles from every possible angle and to build a truly magnificent pair of arms. You'll enjoy dumbell training—I know I do—and you'll get real results on your dumbell days.

Fifty Bar Bell Exercises

To supplement the list of 101 dumbell exercises I have compiled will be the following, at least a hundred additional exercises, which principally involve the arms. With bar bells we can practice the following result-producing exercises:

1.   Front curl.

2.   Back curl.

3.   Curl with one arm front, the other back, reversing the position of the hands at times.

4.   Upright rowing motion.

5.   Leaning over rowing motion.

6.   Continental press.

7.   Military or regular press.

8.   Press behind neck.

9.   Clean.

10.   Jerk.

11.   Continental and jerk behind neck.

12.   Two hands regular snatch.

13.   Dead hang snatch. This movement can be practiced in a variety of forms: With legs straight and only the action of the back and arms. Bending the back and legs, permitting the bar to lower until it nearly touches the floor, then pulling it rather slowly to a height which permits getting under the bell. And with a lighter weight, the pulling up of the weight entirely with the arms and shoulders, back and legs straight and then splitting under the bar to fix it at arm's length.

14.   Right hand side press.

15. Left hand side press.

16. Left hand military press.

17. Right hand military press.

18. Right hand snatch.

19. Left hand snatch.

20. Right hand clean.

21. Left hand clean.

22. Left hand jerk.

23. Right hand jerk.

24. Floor press.

25. Press on box or bench.

26. Two arm pull over. Principally involves the Latissimus and the Pectorals but provides plenty of developmental value for the arms.

27. Dead lift, pulling weight as high as possible. The handling of really heavy poundages such as this movement permits will toughen, enlarge and strengthen all the muscles, tendons, ligaments and attachments of the arm.

28. Pressing in wrestler's bridge position.

29. Starting the bar with weight overhead, lower it to near the floor and on up to overhead at the other side of the body with a swinging motion. As you get the rhythm of this particular movement you will find that the arms have plenty of work to do.

30. Holding the bar bell behind back, leaning the trunk front, and developing the Triceps while straightening the arm.

31.   Sitting upon a chair, elbows resting upon the thighs, raising and lowering the bar bell with wrist action alone to develop the forearm.

32.   Regular curl while leaning forward with upper body parallel to floor. No supporting, action of the elbows against the body is possible in this and the movement to follow; it is purely a muscle developing exercise and brings good results.

33.   Back hand curl while leaning.

34.   Holding bar bell behind back. Perform a motion similar to the upright rowing motion. This will involve the arms in a new and different manner.

35.   Pressing the weight overhead while standing with the elbows front and high.

36.   A somewhat similar movement, this time curling the weight to the shoulders, holding the knuckles up at shoulders, the elbows extended to the front, pressing the weight overhead solely by back hand arm action.

37.   Regular curl and the opposite press without changing the position of the hands. Differs from No. 35 in the fact that the elbows are not moved in No. 35 and No. 37 is performed as a regular press except that the knuckles are front instead of the palms.

38.   An alternate movement of the arms, curling one arm as the other remains extended, then reversing. Can be done with the regular or back hand style. Imparts a somewhat different muscular effect.

39.   Two hands press while sitting upon a chair.

40.   A motion somewhat similar to the upright rowing motion except that the weight is pulled to arm's length overhead. Do not turn the wrists until you are forced to do so at the height of the pull.

41.   A combination exercise. Front curl, regular press and regular rowing.

42.   A directly opposite combination. Back curl, press behind neck and upright rowing motion.

43.   A combination exercise. Start with the weight at arm's length overhead. Lower the bell to the floor, skip the feet back into the floor dip position. Dip until chest touches the bar. then bring feet back to original position. Pull and press the weight to arm's length overhead, and repeat until tired or the desired number of counts have been attained. Considerable strength is required to prevent the bar from rolling while dipping and of course this adds to the results obtained.

44.   In the supine position upon box, extend the arms so that the bar bell rests upon thighs. With a motion similar to the back hand curl, bring the bar to the chest with as little elbow movement as possible, then press the weight to straight arm's length back of head. You can continue the movement

back to the thighs in the same manner, or vary it, returning as in the two hands pull over.

45.   A twisting press. Pressing the weight overhead as the body is twisted first far to the left and then far to the right.

46.   A somewhat different form of swing. Bend down, placing the bar against the floor to the left of the left foot. Raise the bar to arm's length overhead and down to the right of the right foot—this with a semicircular motion. Continue this circular movement until the desired number of counts are reached.

47.   With a bar bell only moderate in length. Starting with the knuckles up—bar against the thighs—extend it to arm's length in front of the body. Do not just swing it up.

206

Rather draw it up nearly to shoulder height in somewhat similar fashion as in the rowing motion, then press it to arm's length in front of the body. Return to the thigh position and continue the exercise in the same manner until the desired number of counts are attained.

48.   Lying face down upon bench. Regular curl, curling weights to height of head. Can be performed in back hand style as well.

49.   Bench press with the hands very wide apart. Involves the muscles from an entirely different angle.

50.   Back hand curl and press with hands together at the bar. A very difficult style. You'll find that it brings you results when you feel the muscles after a few movements.

This list contains fifty good exercises, many of them tried and proven—exercises which have long been a part of York bar bell courses 1, 2, 3, 4, 5 and 6. But many of them are the pet exercises of strength champions and perfect men who train in the York Bar Bell Gym. Some of them are entirely original, few of them little known—plenty of variety. Plenty of muscle, too, will result by choosing your bar bell arm development exercises from this group.

Fifty Additional Exercises

In hand balancing there are many good, result-producing movements—not as many as with apparatus which permits a greater range of movement, but there are many good ones in this list.

1.   Press up into a hand stand.

2.   Walking upon the hands.

3.   One hand stand for the more advanced balancers.

4.   And hopping on one hand for those who become really skillful. This movement has often been done and it results in the most terrific development you have ever seen of the hands, wrists, forearms and Triceps especially.

5.   Tiger bends.

6.   Pressing exercises either from the hand stand position or on boxes with the feet against a wall.

7.   Balancing upon all the fingers.

8.   Lifting the little fingers, the second fingers and if you are really good you'll get as far as Bob Jones with his thumb balance upon Indian Clubs, or with one finger and two thumbs as performed by Val de Genaro.

9.   Coming down stairs with a jumping action while walking upon the hands.

10.   Jumping over boxes, bench or humans, landing upon the hands and retaining a balance.

GOOD EXERCISES WITH CABLES

11.   Front press.

12.   Back press.

13.   Pressing overhead with one arm, holding the other end of the cable with extended arm back of body.

14.   One hand curl, front and back, left.

15.   Right hand curl, front and back.

16.   Two hands curl, palms up.

17.   Two hands curl, knuckles up.

18.   Rowing motion, upright position with stirrups.

19.   Spreading arms to side while leaning.

20.   Rowing motion while cables are held by the feet. This movement is usually performed by stretching the center of the cables over the bottoms of the feet. There is as much resistance as you could wish for in this movement and the arms will have plenty of work to do.

21.   Raise to side. A very good Deltoid developer but benefits the arm, too, owing to its attachment with the shoulder muscles.

22.   Archer's movement. Practiced with first the right and then the left arm extended.

23.   Press across back, starting with one hand straight and pressing out the other. Reverse, starting first with the left arm straight, the right pressing, then the right straight, the left pressing.

24.   Hold arms at shoulders, cable back of neck, forearms in gooseneck position. Stretch cable by straightening the forearms until the arm is fully extended at sides.

25.   A somewhat similar movement except that the entire arm is involved. Instead of just straightening the arms by moving the forearm, start with the upper arm against the body and press them out, holding the hands and wrists in the gooseneck position.

26.   Pull arms down from overhead, stretching cables at shoulder height. The best Latissimus developer known, but one which aids the development of the arm owing to the attachments of the Latissimus to the upper arm.

27.   Spread arms from front at shoulder height, keeping them straight throughout.

28.   Raise the arms in front of body from a beginning, ex

tended down with cables across thigh, to the point where they are extended overhead. Keep arms straight throughout.

29.   A somewhat similar movement behind back. Knuckles up, raise the arms, stretching the cables as far as your muscles will permit.

30.   Starting with the arms extended to the front, backs of hands toward each other, extend the arms to the side at shoulder height. Keep arms straight throughout.

GIANT CRUSHER GRIP EXERCISES

31.   Close grips with arms in front of chest, handles down.

32.   A somewhat similar movement except that the handles of the Giant Crusher are held up and the range of exertion of the arms is up instead of down.

33.   Close the grip at arm's length in front of the body, hands up.

34.   Directly opposite. Close grip with arms in front of body, hands down.

35.   Close the grip in back of head.

36.   Hold the hands between the knees and partly with arm pressure and partly with leg pressure close the grip. You can exert as much or as little pressure as desired with your arms. It brings the Sartorius group of muscles of the

leg into play when practiced as a leg developing exercise. One of the particularly hard muscles to reach.

37.   Holding the Crusher Grip at the left side, lower arm stationary. Close the Crusher with a downward movement of the upper arm.

38.   The same movement on the other side.

39.   Holding the Crusher at floor level, hold with upper arm and pull up with the left. The first exercise performed on the left side.

40.   A similar movement on the right side of body.

EXERCISES WITH THE IRON SHOE

41.   Pull apart at chest level.

42.   Pull apart back of head.

43.   Pull apart, one hand straight in front.

44.   Pull apart, one hand at floor level.

45.   Pull apart, holding Shoe in back of body.

FREE HAND EXERCISE

46.   Chinning, front, back, one hand.

47.   Rope climbing.

48.   Floor dip, two hands.

49.   Floor dip, one hand.

50.   Arm resistance exercises as mentioned in another chapter.

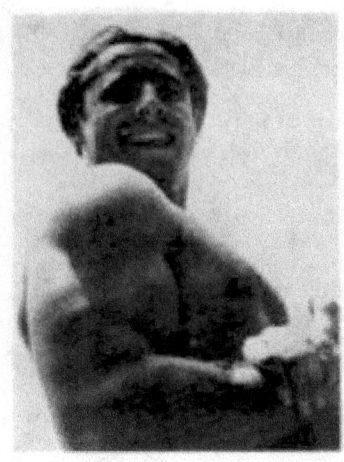

Steve Stanko, holder of the U. S. Heavy-weight Lifting Records.